T0321656

Electrical Safety Code Manual

Electrical Safety Code Manual

A Plain Language Guide to National Electrical Code, OSHA, and NFPA 70E

Kimberley Keller

AMSTERDAM • BOSTON • HEIDELBERG • LONDON
NEW YORK • OXFORD • PARIS • SAN DIEGO
SAN FRANCISCO • SINGAPORE • SYDNEY • TOKYO
Butterworth-Heinemann is an imprint of Elsevier

ELSEVIER

Butterworth-Heinemann is an imprint of Elsevier
30 Corporate Drive, Suite 400, Burlington, MA 01803, USA
The Boulevard, Langford Lane, Kidlington, Oxford, OX5 1GB, UK

Notices

Knowledge and best practice in this field are constantly changing. As new research and experience broaden our understanding, changes in research methods, professional practices, or medical treatment may become necessary.

Practitioners and researchers must always rely on their own experience and knowledge in evaluating and using any information, methods, compounds, or experiments described herein. In using such information or methods they should be mindful of their own safety and the safety of others, including parties for whom they have a professional responsibility.

To the fullest extent of the law, neither the Publisher nor the authors, contributors, or editors, assume any liability for any injury and/or damage to persons or property as a matter of products liability, negligence or otherwise, or from any use or operation of any methods, products, instructions, or ideas contained in the material herein.

Library of Congress Cataloging-in-Publication Data
Keller, K. J. (Kimberley J.)
    Electrical safety code manual: a plain language guide to National electrical code, OSHA, and NFPA 70E / Kimberley Keller.
        p. cm.
    Includes bibliographical references and index.
    ISBN 978-1-85617-654-5 (alk. paper)
    1. Electrical engineering–Safety measures. 2. Industrial safety. 3. Electrical engineering–Standards–United States. 4. Electric apparatus and appliances–Safety measures. I. Title.
    TK152.K428 2010
    621.319′240289–dc22   2009052175

British Library Cataloguing-in-Publication Data
A catalogue record for this book is available from the British Library.

For information on all Butterworth–Heinemann publications
visit our Web site at www.elsevierdirect.com

Printed in the United States of America
10 11 12 13 14   10 9 8 7 6 5 4 3 2 1

Contents

Preface

We have been manipulating power since the time of the caveman. About half a million years ago, mankind mastered fire. The energy source was easy, even for them, to understand; if you touched it, you would get burned. A 1000 years later, the ancient Greeks discovered that rubbing fur on amber caused a spark of energy, and by the seventeenth century, the differentiation between positive and negative currents was discovered. In the year 1600, an English physician named William Gilbert coined the term *electric*, from the Greek *elektron*, to identify the force that certain substances exert when rubbed against each other. It was a great leap forward from rubbing two sticks together to generate enough heat to make fire.

Then, in 1800, an Italian physicist named Alessandro Volta discovered that certain chemical reactions could produce electricity and he created the first transmission of electricity by linking positively-charged and negatively-charged connectors. Volta found that he could force an electrical charge, or voltage, through the connectors. Over time, higher voltages were generated and a new discovery was made; electrical current could cause burns, severe injury, and even death. It could start fires, it could cause materials to arc or explode. It quickly became apparent that electricity had both infinite possibilities for society and unrestrained potential to cause extreme damage. In order for us to be able to survive using electricity, we had to develop a means of safely working with electrical power, wiring, conductors, generators, and other related equipment and components.

Perhaps you have been a licensed electrician for years and maybe you've received a little jolt now and then, but nothing serious. But the reality is that electrical injuries cause about 1000 deaths annually in the United States and are responsible for about 5% of burn center admissions. While you may have escaped serious injury over the years, the fact is that electrical injuries rank as the fifth most common cause of occupational fatalities. The best way for anyone who works with electrical systems to prevent injury to themselves or others, as well as damage to property, is to practice proven electrical safety methods. Electrical safety programs in the workplace not only decrease the incidence of injury, but also protect companies and their employees from the financial ramifications of a work-related accident.

In the case of the electrical industry, safety is critical and the codes and regulations that determine safe practices are both diverse and complicated. Employers, electricians, electrical system designers, inspectors, engineers, and architects must all comply with safety standards listed in the National Electrical Code, OSHA and NFPA 70E. Unfortunately, the publications that list these safety requirements are written in very technically advanced terms and the average person has an extremely difficult time understanding exactly what they need to do to ensure safe installations and working environments.

This book will tie together the various regulations and practices for electrical safety and translate these complicated standards into easy-to-understand terms. Even veteran master electricians will find it informative and gain a new understanding of how to minimize their exposure to possibly injury. After all, you're worth it.

Acknowledgments

Putting together a book about a subject as truly important as safety takes a lot of work, long hours, and a high level of dedication. There have been times when this process has required a great degree of patience from the people closest to me. These people include my son, Adam, who mows the lawn, takes care of the dog, works hauling firewood, shovels snow, and makes the world's best brownies as a treat for me. My daughter, Afton, who stayed focused and determined, graduated magna cum laude with B.S. and B.A. degrees, is now working on her master's degree, and tells me I'm her hero. My life-mate Steve, who brings me coffee, encourages me to keep moving forward, and can always make me laugh. My dad, Bob, who taught me how to think like an engineer, and my mom, Joy, who gave me creativity. These are the people I stay safe for, the ones I work hard for, the ones who make coming home the best part of my day. I hope you take a couple of extra minutes a day to stay safe for the people who care about you.

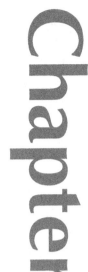

Regulatory Agencies and Organizations
What Are They and What Do They Do?

Chapter Outline

All construction trades come with a degree of physical risk. Early in our country's industrial history tradesman discovered through trial and error which construction methods were the easiest to perform. Unfortunately, easier was not necessarily safer, and many tradesmen were injured or even killed performing their jobs. Over time other factors surfaced, such as the results of poor quality construction methods that lead to the destruction of property. The potential for electricity to start fires, burn, shock, and even kill became quickly apparent and it was obvious that a set of guidelines was needed to reduce the likelihood of damage to both property and people.

1

By the late 1800s, more and more people were depending on electricity to power an ever-increasing number of conveniences from light bulbs to elevators. Installation techniques were based on trial-and-error, experience and best judgment. This left the door open to a multitude of installation techniques, a complete lack of continuity, and a dramatic increase in the number of injuries and fires caused by electricity. Coincidentally, in 1890 Edwin R. Davis, an Auburn Prison electrician, designed the electric chair that utilized 1400 V of direct electrical current for the sole purpose of causing death. Its first use in August of that year was a gruesome example that electricity could kill a person. Between the increasing demand for electricity and the shocking reality of its deadly potential, it is not surprising that the need became apparent for some kind of uniform regulation process for electrical installations. In 1897 the National Fire Protection Association (NFPA) issued the National Electrical Code (NEC), commonly known today as the NEC. Since that time, the NEC has instituted standards designed to protect both people and property from electrical damage. Although the NEC is not itself a U.S. law, it is commonly mandated by state and local laws.

The need for standardized code

The benefit to having one standardized set of regulations is clear. In the U.S., any person, company, or principality can be sued for creating a negligent situation that results in the loss of life or property. Never is the city issuing building permits exempt from this civil liability. Negligence is generally defined as failure to use reasonable care or prudence which results in injury or damage to a person or property. In order to establish reasonable care, uniform standards are needed which establish best practices for safety in trades and industry. A municipality can best avoid lawsuits by focusing on a single source of proven safety codes, and the NEC has become the most widely accepted standard set for electrical requirements. Most states require electrical installations to be inspected for compliance with the standards of the NEC. A failed inspection will cost you time and money to fix and can stop your project in its tracks. Additionally, a majority of states also base their licensing programs and mandatory examinations on the diverse conditions and methods covered in the NEC. The bottom line for an electrician is that if you don't know the NEC standards, your livelihood will ultimately be affected.

The national electrical code

The NEC establishes regulations for the installation of electrical conductors, equipment, raceways, and signaling and communications systems. The code covers public and private premises including homes, buildings and structures, mobile homes, recreational vehicles, and floating buildings. Installation locations include yards, parking lots, carnivals, and industrial substations. The NEC also sets standards for the installation of conductors and equipment that connect to electricity supplies, and installations used by electrical utilities such as office buildings, garages, warehouses, machine shops, recreational buildings, and other structures that are not an integral part of generating plants, substations, or control centers (Figure 1.1).

DEFINITIONS

• ARTICLE – a segment of the Code focused on a specifc topic. Artides are numbered and divided by Sections numbered as subsets. Example: Article 100, Section 100.1

• CODE – An extensive compilation of provisions covering broad subject matter or that is suitable for adoption into law independently of other codes and standards.

• FPN – Abbreviation for Fine-Print Note which supplements an Article's rules. FPNs are not requirements and are for information purposes only.

• MANDITORY – A provision of the NEC that must be followed by law. Mandatory rules are marked by the word "shall."

• STANDARD – A document that contains only mandatory provisons which use the work "shall" to indicate requirements and that is in a form generally suitable for mandatory reference by another standard or code, or that is for adoption into law. Nonmandatory provisions are located in the appendix, footnotes, or fine-print note and are not considered a part of the requirements of a standard.

Figure 1.1 Key NEC Terms.

NFPA's Committee on the NEC consists of 20 code-making panels and a technical committee that develops and updates the NEC. In order to draw on the collective wisdom of the international community, the code panels have members from countries other than the United States, as well as members of the world's leading professional association for the advancement of technology which is the Institute of Electrical and Electronics Engineers, Inc. (IEEE). The NEC is formally identified as ANSI/NFPA 70 and is approved as an American national standard by the American National Standards Institute (ANSI). Even with it setting minimum standards, the NEC is the least amended model code. Changes to the code are typically made to allow for new technologies or to combine or clarify existing standards.

Composed of an introduction, nine chapters, annexes A through G, and an index, the NEC groups standards in a logical progression. The introduction explains the purpose and general rules for overall electrical safety and enforcement. Safeguarding people and property from hazards arising from the use of electricity is the primary purpose of the NEC. Distinctions are made between establishing safety provisions included in the NEC and additional effort that might be necessary for installations to be efficient, convenient, or adequate for good service or future expansion. In this way, the code establishes a baseline for installation practices, while making clear that it is not intended to be a design specification or instruction manual (Figure 1.2).

Article 90 of the NEC describes what the code does and does not cover, how it is arranged, and distinguishes between mandatory rules, permissive rules, and explanatory material. Governmental agencies that regulate construction processes, such as the municipality in which a project takes place, are identified as the authority having jurisdiction (AHJ) and are given a degree of enforcement flexibility by the code. Additionally, products that are listed, such as underwriters listed (UL) can be assumed to be adequate for their stated purpose and do not have to be inspected again, except for alterations or damage.

The first four chapters cover definitions and rules for installations for voltages, connections, markings, circuits, and circuit protection; however, voltage drop requirements are not covered. Standards

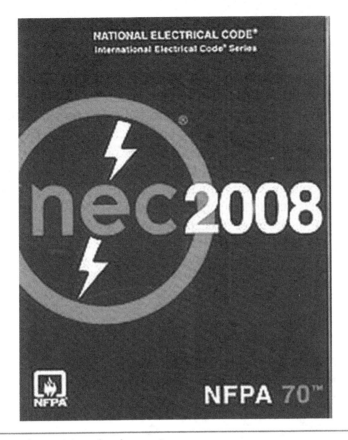

Figure 1.2 The NEC is updated every 3 years.

for methods and materials for wiring, devices, conductors, cables, as well as general-purpose equipment including cords, receptacles, switches, and heaters are also outlined in the first four chapters of the NEC.

The next three chapters focus on special occupancies, ranging from multiple-family units to high risk installations, as well as specific equipment such as signs and machinery, and special conditions including emergency systems and alarms. Chapter 8 is dedicated to additional requirements for communications systems and Chapter 9 is comprised of tables that further clarify requirements for conductors, cables, and conduit properties. The appendix provides calculations, examples, and explanations of implementation of code articles, such as how many wires fit in a conduit.

In addition to the NEC book, an NEC Handbook is published which is the equivalent of an annotated edition of the NEC. The handbook offers insights and explanations of new and more difficult articles and provides a guide to interpreting and applying current code requirements to various types of electrical installations. Expert commentary explains the rationale behind the standards and offers practical, hands-on advice on how to comply with regulations. It contains color-coded commentary that is set apart from the mandatory NEC provisions and summaries of key changes in each article (Figure 1.3).

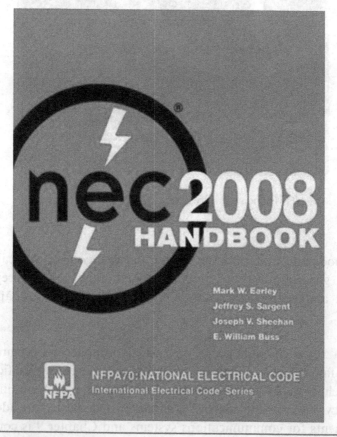

Figure 1.3 The NEC Handbook.

National fire protection association

The NEC is only one of several standardized safety volumes published by the NFPA. The NFPA is a U.S. organization developed to create and maintain minimum standards and requirements for fire prevention, fire suppression, training, and other life-safety codes. All types of subjects are covered from building codes, emergency response methods, and investigations, to personal protective equipment (PPE) for both electrical tradesmen and firefighters. Publications are numbered for identification and include the following:

■ NFPA 70—National Electrical Code

■ NFPA 70B—Recommended Practice for Electrical Equipment Maintenance

■ NFPA 70E—Standard for Electrical Safety in the Workplace

■ NFPA 72—National Fire Alarm Code

■ NFPA 79—Restriction of Access to Hazardous Energy

■ NFPA 101—Life Safety Code

■ NFPA 704—Standard System for the Identification of the Hazards of Materials for Emergency Response

■ NFPA 853—Standard for the Installation of Stationary Fuel Cell Power Systems

■ NFPA 921—Guide for Fire and Explosion Investigations

Fees received from these technical manuals and other material finance the NFPA.

The NFPA was originally formed in 1896 by a group of insurance representatives who thought it prudent to establish standards for the emerging market of fire sprinkler systems. Within a year, the NFPA's focus broadened to the development of regulations for fire protection in another fast-growing technology—building electrical systems. From there it developed codes for all aspects of building design and construction.

Its original membership of insurance underwriters had no direct experience or representation from the industries the NFPA sought to regulate, but this changed in 1904 when representatives from other industries were encouraged to participate in the development of the standards created by the association. In 1905, the New York City Fire Department became the first fire department to be represented in the NFPA. The modern NFPA includes representatives from fire departments, insurance companies, manufacturing associations, unions, trade organizations, engineers, and average citizens. Most of our current fire-related safety laws are developed from research conducted by this organization.

Headquartered in Quincy, Massachusetts, today's NFPA oversees the development and revision of over 300 codes and standards. The association's standards and codes are nationally accepted as a professional standard, and are recognized by many courts as the minimum requirements for safety.

Birth of a code or standard

The NFPA Board of Directors is in charge of all activities of the NFPA, and it issues all rules and regulations that govern the development of NFPA codes and standards. A standards council is appointed by the board to oversee the association's codes and standards development activities, administer the rules and regulations, and act as an appeals body. Additionally, there are over 250 code making panels and technical committees that are responsible for developing and revising NFPA codes and standards. In addition to acting on their own proposed changes, these technical committees and panels also review proposed changes to NFPA documents. Any interested party can submit these.

Committees and panels are organized into projects with an assigned scope of activities. Depending on the subject involved, a project can develop one code or standard or a group of related codes and standards, and the project may consist of a single technical committee or multiple committees and code making panels. A technical correlating committee resolves any conflicts or concerns and ensures consistency coordinates the committees and panels.

National electrical safety code

The IEEE, administers the National Electrical Safety Code (NESC®) that sets the ground rules for practical safety codes for people involved in the installation, operation, or maintenance of electric supply and communication lines and equipment. At first glance, this might seem like a duplication of material covered in the NEC; however, each code covers uniquely different aspects of electrical installations. While the NEC is focused on hazards arising from the use of electricity in buildings and structures, the NESC is designed to bring consistency and safety to the design, construction, operation, and use of electric supply and communication installations. Excluded from the standards covered by the NESC are installations in mines, ships, railway rolling equipment, aircraft, automotive equipment, and utilization wiring.

From 1973 to 1993, the NESC was revised every 3 years. Beginning with the 2002 edition, the NESC began issuing updated publications every 5 years, with the next scheduled revision due in 2012. The NESC is made up of subcommittees that are responsible for the content of the NESC. Subcommittee section assignments are as follows:

- Subcommittee 1—Coordination (Sections 1, 2, and 3; coordination between technical subcommittees)

- Subcommittee 2—Grounding Methods (Section 9)

- Subcommittee 3—Electric Supply Stations (Sections 10-19)

- Subcommittee 4—Overhead Lines—Clearances (Sections 20-23)

- Subcommittee 5—Overhead Lines—Strength and Loading (Sections 24-27)

- Subcommittee 7—Underground Lines (Sections 30-39)

- Subcommittee 8—Work Rules (Sections 40-43)

As with the NEC, the NESC is written as a voluntary standard. However, some editions and some parts of the code have been adopted, with and without changes, by some state and local jurisdictional authorities. You can determine the legal status of the NESC in any particular state or locality by contacting the AHJ in your area.

American national standards institute

The ANSI is a nonprofit organization that oversees the development of voluntary standards for products, services, processes, systems, and personnel in the United States. The organization also coordinates U.S. standards with international standards so that American products can be used worldwide. For example, standards make sure that people who own cameras can find the film they need for them anywhere around the globe.

The ANSI mission is to enhance the global competitiveness of U.S. business and the U.S. quality of life by promoting and facilitating conformity and voluntary consensus standards and maintaining their integrity.

ANSI accredits standards that ensure consistency among the characteristics and performance of products, that people use the same definitions and terms regarding materials, and that products are tested the same way. ANSI also accredits organizations that certify products or personnel in accordance with requirements that are defined in international standards.

The institute is like the umbrella that covers thousands of guidelines that directly impact businesses in almost every sector. Everything from construction equipment, to dairy standards, to energy distribution, and electrical materials is affected. ANSI is also actively engaged in accrediting programs that assess conformance to standards, including globally recognized programs such as the ISO 9000 Quality Management and ISO 14,000 Environmental Systems.

The ANSI has served as administrator and coordinator of the United States private sector voluntary standardization system since 1918. It was founded by five engineering societies and three government agencies. Today, the Institute represents the interests of its nearly 1000 company, organization, government agency, institutional, and international members through its headquarters in Washington, D.C.

Accreditation by ANSI signifies that a procedure meets the Institute's essential requirements for openness, balance, consensus, and due process safeguards. For this reason, American National Standards are referred to as "open" standards. In this context, open refers to a process that is used by a recognized organization for developing and approving a standard. The Institute's definition of "open" basically refers to a collaborative, balanced, and consensus-based approval process. The criteria used to develop these open standards balance the interests of those who will implement the standard with the interests and voluntary cooperation of those who own property or use rights that are essential to or affected by the standard. For this reason, ANSI standards are required to undergo public reviews. In addition to facilitating the creation of standards in our country, ANSI promotes the use of U.S. standards internationally and advocates U.S. policy and technical positions in international and regional standards organizations (Figure 1.4).

OCCUPATIONAL SAFETY AND HEALTH ASSOCIATION (OSHA)

The Occupational Safety and Health Administration (OSHA) is a United States Department of Labor agency. It was originally created by Congress under the Occupational Safety and Health Act, signed by President Richard M. Nixon on December 29, 1970. Unlike other organizations such as NESC or ANSI, OSHA is not publically run, but is comprised of private company representatives. OSHA's statutory authority extends to non-governmental workplaces where there are employees. The Occupational Safety and Health Act allows states to develop their own approved plans as long as they cover public sector employees and provide protection that is equivalent to the requirements outlined by federal OSHA regulations. The mission of OSHA is to prevent work-related injuries, illnesses, and deaths by issuing and enforcing standards for workplace safety and health, providing training, outreach, and education, establishing partnerships, and encouraging continual improvement in workplace safety and health. This means this agency oversees regulations that affect both employers and employees.

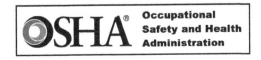

Figure 1.4 The Occupational Safety and Health Administration publishes regulations by which safety in the workplace are measured.

OSHA's Voluntary Protection Program (VPP) encourages voluntary programs and partnerships with industry. In the VPP, management, labor, and OSHA establish cooperative relationships at workplaces that have implemented a comprehensive safety and health management system. Approval into VPP is OSHA's official recognition of the outstanding efforts of employers and employees for demonstrated exemplary occupational safety and health. It is sometimes believed that the agency promotes only "voluntary compliance" when, in fact, all employers are required by law to comply with all the rules published under the Occupational Safety and Health Act of 1970. Non-compliance results in citations and fines, which in turn affect an employer's MOD rating, insurance premiums, and even its ability to qualify to bid on some large-scale projects (Figure 1.5).

OSHA is only able to pursue a criminal penalty when a willful violation of an OSHA standard results in the death of a worker. However, if a project is found to be in violation of OSHA standards, work cannot continue until the infraction has been rectified and compliance is approved by an OSHA inspection. All of these conditions may make OSHA seem like a big, bad monster to be feared and loathed. In reality, OSHA has dedicated years to analyzing and issuing regulations to protect and further workplace health. For example, in 2001 OSHA issued ergonomic specific guidelines based on years of study. Ergonomic injuries, also known as musculoskeletal injuries, which include back injuries and carpal tunnel syndrome, account for one-third of all serious injuries suffered by American workers.

WHAT IS A MOD?

An experience modifer or "MOD" is the actual number of losses over the predicted number of losses which gives you a number which is usually between 0.10 and 1.99. In regards to Workers Compensation, your dollar losses are a percentage of what the expected dollar losses would be for employers with your type of trade exposure. A low MOD will result in a reduction in an employer's Workers Compensation premiums; however, injury claims and OSHA citations can cause a MOD greater than 1.00 and result in high premium or assessment costs.

Figure 1.5 MOD rates can be higher for companies with OSHA citations.

OSHA offers a free consultation service for small business owners, including help in identifying workplace hazards and establishing or improving safety and health management systems across the company.

Some of the most common workplace hazards and injuries identified by OSHA include:

- Slips, trips, and falls

- Strains and sprains

- Chemical exposure

- Burns and cuts

- Eye injuries

- Hearing loss

- Electrocution

- Tool and machinery malfunctions

As a result of identifying these hazards, several changes in overall industrial safety regulations have been initiated by OSHA, including the following:

- *Guards on all moving parts:* Includes guards to prevent inadvertent contact with most moving parts that are accessible in the normal course of operation. With OSHA, the use of guards was expanded to cover essentially all parts where contact is possible.

- *Permissible exposure limits (PEL):* Identifies the maximum safe concentrations of chemicals and dusts.

- *Personal protective equipment:* Focuses on the use of respirators, gloves, coveralls, hardhats, and other protective equipment when handling or working with or around hazardous materials, including electricity.

- *Lockout/tagout:* Covers requirements for locking out energy sources by securing them in an "off" condition when performing repairs or maintenance.

- *Confined space:* Specific requirements for air sampling and the use of a "buddy system" when working inside tanks, manholes, pits, bins, and similar enclosed areas.

- *Process safety management:* Designed to reduce large scale industrial accidents.

- *Bloodborne pathogen:* Protects health care and other workers from being exposed to bloodborne pathogens such as Hepatitis B and HIV.

- *Excavations and trenches:* OSHA regulations specify that employees working 5 feet deep or more in trenches and excavations must be provided with safeguards in addition to proper sloping and storage of excavated material in order to prevent collapses and cave-ins.

OSHA encourages companies to recognize and remove hazards from worksites and protect workers from injury, illness, and death. Compliance with OSHA regulations also cultivates informed and alert employees who take responsibility for their own safety, their coworkers' safety, and for workplace safety as a whole.

A little knowledge goes a long way

For the average company or employee, the most difficult part of complying with NEC, OSHA, or other standards is understanding the regulations. The wording in these codes and guidelines is generally very technical and can be more than a little confusing. The good news is that many of the standards parallel one another from one publication to the next, so that once you decipher the requirements, compliance with all of the applicable code is relatively easy.

Ultimately, the primary goal of any company or worker needs to be safety first. Injuries hurt everyone involved. Companies suffer from increased insurance premiums and diminished or lost production from valuable employees. Workers are forced to endure not only pain and recuperation time, but also diminished income and possible long-term disability. Safety codes are the results of years of study, data comparisons, and invaluable contributions from experienced tradesmen, businesses, and industry representatives. These regulations exist to protect you. Sometimes you may think they are inconvenient or a burden, but if you abide by them, hopefully you will never have to experience the pain and suffering of a workplace injury (Figure 1.00).

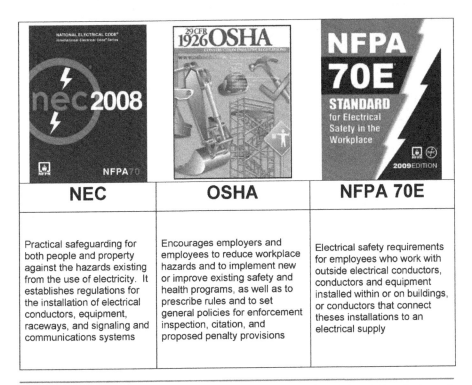

NEC	OSHA	NFPA 70E
Practical safeguarding for both people and property against the hazards existing from the use of electricity. It establishes regulations for the installation of electrical conductors, equipment, raceways, and signaling and communications systems	Encourages employers and employees to reduce workplace hazards and to implement new or improve existing safety and health programs, as well as to prescribe rules and to set general policies for enforcement inspection, citation, and proposed penalty provisions	Electrical safety requirements for employees who work with outside electrical conductors, conductors and equipment installed within or on buildings, or conductors that connect theses installations to an electrical supply

Figure 1.00   The three central electricals safaty texts are the National Electrical coad, OSHA, and NFPA 70E.

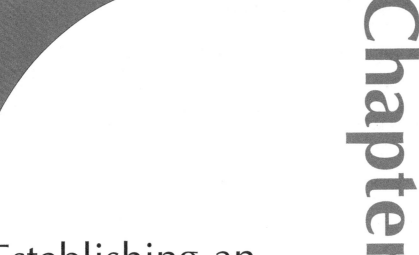

Establishing an Effective Electrical Safety Program

Chapter 2

OSHA has concluded that there are several factors that can combine to reduce the extent and severity of work-related injuries and illnesses. An effective written safety program, accident prevention plans, and

17

Doi: 10.1016/B978-1-85617-654-5.00002-9

management of worker safety and health protection are key elements to maintaining worker health on the job. One of the most important priorities of supervisors and managers should be to send their employees home in as good a condition as when they arrived at work. This means leaving work free from injuries or illnesses due to work-related incidents.

In addition to ensuring a safer workplace, thorough safety programs and accident prevention plans should be designed to decrease workplace injuries and illnesses, reduce lost time, increase compliance with the law and, by doing so, lower insurance costs. When an employer places emphasis on effective safety programs, employee morale, commitment, and trust will also increase. Having a company that is recognized for its good safety performance can also help in recruiting and retaining highly skilled and talented individuals. Additionally, these programs can improve a company's public image, which is extremely important in today's competitive workplace. No company can afford to be perceived as unsafe, and companies should strive to represent good stewardship to the communities they service and to society as a whole.

Measuring the results of workplace safety programs is essential to employers and employees because both gain confidence that changes can and will be made that result in a safer workplace. Employee feedback is vital to the on-going evolution and long-term success of an effective safety program.

Basic components of a comprehensive safety program and accident prevention plan include a number of key elements, such as:

- Clearly established safety program goals and objectives, including a mission statement by owners or management stating that safety is the company's primary priority

- Implementation description with actions, responsibilities, and time-frames
  - Written safety policies and procedures
  - A description of unacceptable practices or behaviors and disciplinary consequences

- Regular communications, education, training, and safety meetings

- A workplace hazard safety analysis process

- Effective safety performance measures

- On-going evaluations, safety audits, and job safety inspections

- Corrective action process to identify safety hazards or deficiencies

- Documentation and record keeping process

- Employment related medical requirements

- A process for handling an accident or illness

- Employee assistance program

Safety program goals

What is the rational behind having a safety program? The primary purpose is to ensure that workers go home with the same level of health and well-being that they came to work possessing. A work-related injury is costly on both the human level as well as financially. Far too many workers don't take seriously the possibility of being hurt while they are at work. They figure they are pretty careful, and assume that their experience in the trade is enough to keep them safe. If you were to ask average employees what they think about adhering to a mandatory safety program, they would probably say that they wear a hardhat and maybe safety glasses now and then and that is enough of an inconvenience to deal with. Safety programs are implemented to protect the employer and the employee. Employers can control insurance expenses and operating costs more effectively when their employees are healthy, but why are safety protocols so important to employees?

Here is an example. Maybe you are married with a couple of kids, a mortgage, a truck payment, and some credit card bills; in other words you are an average American. You relay on your weekly level of pay to meet your bills and support your family. Now let's look at a common scenario that results from a typical construction injury: a trip, slip, or fall.

You are headed out to your truck or construction trailer with another employee to get some material while another guy is drilling through a wall to run wire. His cord is stretched across the floor and plugged into an extension cord. You're talking to your co-worker about last night's football game as you walk toward the building exit. You're looking at your buddy, not at the floor, you trip over the extension cord, and "bam" you fall sideways on your knees all disheveled on the concrete floor. No big deal, right? Wrong. This kind of impact with a hard surface can cause the same kind of damage to your knees as a football player hitting the ground during a tackle. How often have you watched one of those guys, who are heavily padded, get up limping as they head toward the sideline. Then they are out of the game because they damaged the ligaments in their knee.

But you are a seasoned tradesman, and you figure it's no big deal. So instead of reporting your fall, you just make light of it, or curse a few times at your drill-wheedling coworker and hobble about your business for the rest of the day with one knee making an annoying popping sound. Probably the last thing you are thinking about is that, just like a downed football player, you may have a soft-tissue injury. Tendon or ligament damage like this can require corrective surgery, but you might not even realize the extent of your injury until the next morning when you get out of bed and realize you can't put any weight on one leg.

Now you have to call in to the office and tell them you fell on the job the day before. The safety manager or human resource director has to get an appointment for you with the company-approved doctor. Yes, the company doctor because you were hurt on the job and now your employer is in charge of your care. The doctor can't see you until the end of the day, so you are already missing a day of work. You get to your appointment where they do an X-ray and tell you that you've torn your anterior cruciate ligament (ACL) (Figure 2.1).

Now, not only are you in pain, but you need to have corrective surgery and you are out of work on workers' compensation. People who have never been injured on the job are often not aware that workers' compensation does not reimburse your lost time at 100% of your normal wage. So, not only are you uncomfortable, but you are not bringing

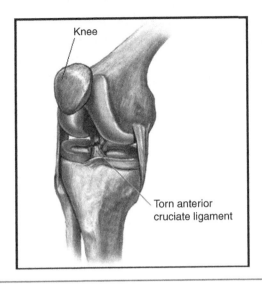

Knee

Torn anterior
cruciate ligament

Figure 2.1 A torn ACL requires surgical repair, several weeks of recovery, and physical therapy.

home the kind of money you would have made if you had not been hurt. To top it off, that mortgage payment and the rest of your bills are all still due regardless of the fact that you have less money. Your employer has to pull another worker off of a different job to do your work while you're out, and has to report your lost time which goes against the company's loss rating. The bottom line is that everyone loses. All of this is from a simple trip and fall accident. Imagine if this were a more seriously debilitating injury, such as a fall from a ladder that resulted in a ruptured disc or an electrical shock that landed you in the intensive care unit of a hospital with third degree burns and permanent damage to your heart.

Safety manuals

The most effective way to communicate a company safety plan is through a written safety manual. This document should be distributed to employees when they are initially hired and should include a separate acceptance page. Once a new hire has read the manual, they need to sign the acceptance page and return it to their employer to signify that they understand the company's safety policies and expectations.

Companies may periodically update their manuals based on experience, changes in policies, or insurance carrier contact information. When this occurs, revised manuals need to be distributed to all employees and a new acceptance page should be signed and returned to management.

A safety manual outlines the safe practice expectations of a company. A company's employee work performance assessment can include adherence to company safety requirements to encourage safe work ethics and diminish injuries.

Elements of a safety handbook

A comprehensive safety handbook begins with a mission statement, signed by management, which sets the tone of the manual by demonstrating that the employer values the well-being of its employees (Figure 2.2).

It is helpful to include a table of contents at the beginning of a safety manual to facilitate quick reference to various safety topics. The first section should outline the expectations of employees with regards to their general safety responsibilities, and timeframes for implementation. For example, "All employees will adhere to the safety requirements outlined in this manual beginning on their first day of employment."

MISSION STATEMENT

Protecting the health and safety of all our employees is the primary concern of all of owners/management of *Company Name*. We strive to achieve and maintain this goal through the implementation of a comprehensive and effective workplace health and safety plan that endeavors to eliminate unsafe conditions and minimize the impact of hazardous situations. We believe that such a program will benefit both the company and employees by reducing illness and injury to personnel, preventing property damage, and encouraging timely, consistent project completion. Our primary priority is to make every reasonable effort to promote, create, and maintain a safe and healthful environment so that employees will leave work in the same healthy condition in which they reported for work. This goal can only be realized by adherence to the basic safety principles outlined in this manual along with sound management practices, and compliance with applicable federal, state, and local codes, laws, and standards.

Figure 2.2 A typical safety manual mission statement.

The bulk of the safety guide should detail the company's safety policies and procedures. Topics should include the use of tools, company vehicles and equipment, any smoking policies, utilization of personal protection equipment, hazardous material handling, and an outline of how to report an injury or illness. Descriptions of unacceptable practices or behaviors and disciplinary consequences should also be listed. Activities such as harassment, horseplay, drug or alcohol use, intimidation or threatening actions, and failure to properly use tools, equipment, and safety protocols (such as lockout/tagout) should be expressly prohibited and punishable acts. Disciplinary actions can include a probationary period, suspension without pay, or discharge, depending on the number and severity of safety protocol infractions.

In addition to an outline of do's and don'ts, the safety manual should address company procedures for workplace safety such as:

- Regular communications, education, training, and safety meetings
- Mandatory compliance with NFAP and OSHA regulations
- Workplace hazard safety and emergency response plans
- Documentation and record keeping process
- On-going evaluations, safety audits, and job safety inspections
- Corrective action process to identify safety hazards or deficiencies
- Employment related medical requirements
- The process for handing an accident or illness
- Employee assistance program.

Let's examine some of these topics in more detail.

Safety meetings

If you tell your employees that it is time for their regular safety training, you can usually expect to hear a collective groan. This is because most employees view safety trainings as a waste of time. If your training consists of a printed handout, they will just give it a glance and sign off on it, and if you interrupt their work schedule to give a personal presentation, employees often get resentful and agitated that you are wasting their valuable time. So the challenge for any employer is to conduct safety trainings that are both informative and interesting. There is a big difference between mere compliance with safety requirements and true reliance on safe practices. When you have genuine buy-in to corporate safety guidelines, the odds are much greater that no one will have to experience the physical and financial pain of a work-related injury.

There is preaching and then there is actual teaching. Before you can teach anyone about safety you have to find a way to get their attention and respect. When you have their attention, they will hear the message you need to convey, and if you have their respect employees will want to apply what you tell them.

Some companies hold weekly safety talks, while others conduct training once a month. The frequency of safety meetings is not specified by OSHA, rather it is typically a business decision based on the size of a company's workforce and the cost to conduct training. The most successful training is presented to a reasonably sized group of employees, no more than about 20 people at a time. If a company has a massive workforce of hundreds of people, then printed safety training can be supplemented annually or bi-annually with a personal presentation to larger groups of employees.

Workers are not going to listen to you if they don't think you have true experience, so don't think they will respect you just because you have a title of authority. Anyone who is designated to hold safety trainings should strive to develop a working relationship with people. If you learn about your employees and know them by name, they'll have an opportunity to learn about your experience in the trade, and respect will be fostered.

Most workers have the feeling that a safety instructor's job isn't to keep them safe, it's really to save the company money by placing burdensome rules and safety guards everywhere. The general attitude among workers is, "Do you want me to meet my work schedule or waste time worrying about being safe?" The first thing you must convey is that safety guards and requirements are not in place to slow production, they exist because an employer truly cares about its employees as people. If you want your workers to believe you care, then solicit their feedback on ways everyone can reduce potential hazards without slowing down production. Some of the best improvements to safety plans have come from the same people who have to implement safety practices everyday. For example, at the end of any safety training, you could ask employees to write down one suggestion for improving safety on the job. Review the feedback, and if a majority of employees point out similar improvements to a common issue, you can modify your safety policy to include their input. This is proof positive that you respect your employees' opinions, experience, and well-being.

You may still have to drag employees to their safety trainings, unless you entice them with free coffee and donuts or pizza. Once they discover that they are going to "really get something" out of the safety trainings, motivating them to attend should not be difficult. Another way to gain employee respect is to identify a required safety feature, such as steel toed shoes, and then develop a way to help ease the workers' burden while speeding up or keeping production the same. For example, a company can offer to reimburse employees a percentage of the cost of their mandatory steel toed shoes or provide workers with tinted safety glasses that they can take home and use for yard work.

Once employees believe you recognize that their time and efforts are assets to your company, you will have a better chance of conducting a truly effective safety training. To be successful, keep safety trainings simple, interesting, and appropriate. Teach workers techniques that realistically apply to them and their job, and modify and qualify your trainings for the skill level of your workers. For instance, an apprentice electrician may not be qualified to operate a forklift, but they do need to know how to behave around them. You can review general forklift safety at the beginning of a training session and then dismiss helpers and unqualified employees while you review safe operations methods with authorized operators.

Teach information that employees have not already heard a hundred times before, and involve workers with interactive techniques. For example, when I was the safety director for a commercial electrical contractor, we found that a lot of employees were complaining of overall back pain at the end of the day. These were not accident-related injuries, so I decided to do some research on the possible causes. The result was our first training by Fred the Head (Figure 2.3).

Fred the Head was a molded, weighted human head on a 2 feet pole that we borrowed from the outreach department of our workers' compensation company. Fred weighed 12 pounds, the equivalent of the average human head. After introducing Fred to our employees, we passed him around to each training participant and asked them to hold him with one hand for 1 min. The catch was that they had to hold Fred at a 45° angle. Most of our big, burly tradesmen scoffed at the challenge, until they had to hold Fred for themselves. As they found themselves struggling to keep Fred from tipping too far forward, I explained to them that gravity was not their friend. Their wrist was now being exposed to the same type of strain that their backs were enduring from gravity pressure that is three times greater at a 45° angle than it is straight up and down. The experience was designed to encourage workers to avoid bending over if they could make slight modifications to their tasks. For example, employees could sit on a bucket or kneel on a kneepad to install receptacle cover plates instead of bending over for hours to complete the finish work. At the end of the training, and

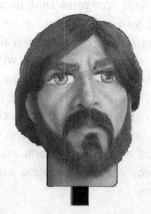

Figure 2.3 Fred the Head hands-on demonstration tools encourage interactive participation during safety trainings.

without ever muttering a word, Fred the Head had inspired our employees to look for ways to avoid back strain, and the incidence of back pain complaints soon reduced dramatically.

Another interactive approach is to break your group into teams and have them answer questions about the safety training in a game-show format. The winning team members could receive an extra work break that day or a company hat. With teaching techniques like this, you encourage your employees to really pay attention to safety topics.

The next step to success is to keep them coming back for more. Consider having a drawing during training for something employees can take home or an item they can use at work that applies to safety. Some examples of giveaways are a home fire extinguisher or smoke alarm when a training is based on emergency response, or a pair of work gloves for use at home when a training covers personal protective equipment (PPE), or just for fun you could have a drawing for a BBQ grill set. On a smaller scale, you could give everyone a coupon for free coffee or pull a name from a hat for a free sub sandwich or a gas gift card. The other element to focus on is the length of time you take out of the workday for safety trainings. Don't spend more than 1 hour for each training unless it's fork truck or respirator training, because you risk losing your audience's attention and allowing them to get bored. It only takes a couple of boring safety trainings to sour your workers' attitude toward participating.

A final suggestion is to get workers involved in safety. Include them on a safety inspection team, a safety improvement team, or let them choose their own training topic for the next meeting. You can even choose one of your employees to be a guest speaker during a training session and share their advice on issues that pertain to their job. A worker who has had a "close-call" on the job, or who has experience that no one else has, for example in working from a bucket-truck, can add a new perspective and flavor to your safety training. Also, encourage your employees to integrate their workplace safety knowledge into safety consciousness at home. Point out that the same hearing protection they gain by wearing ear plugs on the job site can also protect them against hearing loss at home when they are using a chainsaw or power tools.

If you decide to test on training topics, make the tests user friendly. Don't try to trick people, or mark people down for spelling errors or short answers. The goal should be for employees to increase their comprehension and understanding of safety subjects, not to just regurgitate information onto paper. If you decide to use printed safety training handouts, consider printing them with pictures from actual job sites, or use cartoons to add a bit of humor (Figures 2.4 and 2.5).

Training and education

Hands-on training and continuing education based on safe practices help to create and maintain a comprehensive safety program. You can't learn to drive a car on paper and you can't learn to safely operate a bucket-truck, forklift or generator truck by listening to a presenter. Some aspects of safety have to be experienced. Proper use of a respirator, for example, is something that you want your employees to know how to do before they are required to use it in the field. For this reason, companies need to be sure to schedule specific trainings for equipment or procedures that may require certification or qualification. Many companies offer CPR and first aide training to their supervisors and job foremen. These are the individuals who are most likely to be on-site and required to respond and react to an emergency until an ambulance or EMTs can arrive. Most organizations require that individuals who may be required to wear respirators are assessed and approved by a health professional as verification that they are physically capable of operating such safety gear.

> Workers who will be required to wear a respirator should pass a physical examination by a physician to ensure that they do not have any restrictions or impairments that could result in complications from wearing respiration equipment.

Workers who may be required to work in confined spaces should understand the process from start to finish, including the need for a confined space permit or authorization and how to operate any atmospheric testing equipment such as an O_2 meter. These trainings

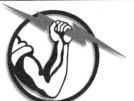

This week's Safety topic:

Material Handling:
Manual and Mechanical

Keller Electrical Contractors
923 Cody Street
Brunswick, ME 04011

SAFETY TRAINING
WEEK #22

Do not lift heavy loads alone, or lift loads beyond your physical capacities. Get help or use mechanical aids. Please note: items that you could easily lift under normal conditions could require you to get help in congested areas or in areas where mobility is hampered.

When handling rough, jagged, or sharp materials, use appropriate gloves or material handing equipment.

Do not pull or tug on material that is "caught" or "hung-up"; it may quickly release and cause an injury.

The following 7 steps are recommended when attempting to lift:

1. Face the load
2. Tuck in you chin
3. Bend your knees
4. Keep your back straight and AVOID TWISTING
5. Keep the load close to your body
6. Establish a firm footing and a solid grip
7. Keep your feet pointed in the direction of the load

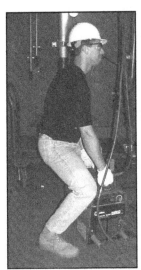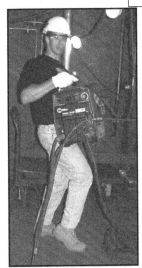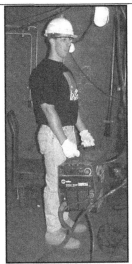

Don't lift from a twisted or awkward position or move to a twisted or awkward position with the material in hand and always get help when you can

Special thanks ot Matt for agreeing to demonstrate this weeks Safety topic

Figure 2.4   Safety topic sheets can include pictures of job sites that your employees have worked on.

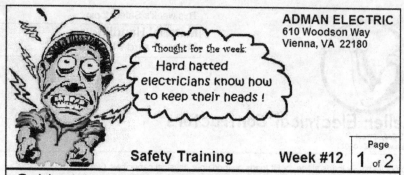

ADMAN ELECTRIC
610 Woodson Way
Vienna, VA 22180

Thought for the week:

Hard hatted
electricians know how
to keep their heads !

Safety Training   **Week #12** | Page **1** of **2**

Subject: Personal Protective Equipment - Your Hard Hat

In 1870, a worker filled his derby hat with paper in hopes that it would protect him against objects that were falling from above on the job he was working. Since that time, with the advancement of technology, engineers have been able to develop stronger and better fitting hats for our protection. When it comes to using this protective equipment, it is important that you understand what responsibilities there are related to inspection, use and care.

HAZARDS TO THE HEAD

It is pretty basic - hard hats are designed to protect against top impact, offer some lateral or side impact protection, and serve as an insulator against electrical shocks. The American National Standards Institute (ANSI) requires that the hard hat must be able to absorb an impact similar to that of a two pound hammer falling two stories. In the actual test, the hard hat rests on a metal head form connected to a transducer that measures the amount of force transmitted through the shell and suspension. An 8-pound ball is dropped from a distance of five feet. On impact, the hard hat shell gives slightly where the ball hits, reducing the initial force and affording the primary protection for the head. Then the suspension's crown assembly takes over by tightening around the head, stretching as it absorbs the energy from the blow within the 1¼ inch clearance between the shell and the suspension. This all takes place in approximately 1/50ᵗʰ of a second.

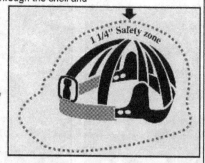

INSPECTION

As you can see, the hard hat is a system made up of different components. If one part of the hard hat is damaged, the entire hard hat system is compromised and you will not be protected. Inspections take on greater importance when you understand how critical they are to your personal safety. Inspect both inside and outside the shell for cracks, nicks, gouges, or cuts. Damage as small as a hairline crack will widen and spread under regular service. If you introduce even minimal impact, the result could be a nasty head or neck injury.

The suspension system should be checked for any signs of wear, such as twisted, cut, torn or frayed straps, loose stitching, or plastic parts with cracks or small breaks. In 4 or 6-point suspension (the number of keys that are engaged in the hard hat's shell), all keys should fit tightly and securely into their respective key slots. Any suspension that shows signs of damage must be removed from service and replaced immediately.

Figure 2.5 You can always add a little humor to your safety trainings.

are on a level beyond standard safety trainings and should be offered annually. Typical training schedules could be as follows:

- *Basic electrical safety awareness:* All employees—upon initial hire and through weekly or monthly safety trainings.

- *Advanced electrical safety:* Employees who work directly with electrical systems from 50 to 600 V, and will therefore are considered qualified or authorized persons—annual training.

- *Specific lockout/tagout training:* Employees who work directly with electrical systems from 50 to 600 V, and will therefore are considered qualified or authorized persons—annual training.

- *Respirator training:* Employees who have been assessed as physically able to work while wearing a respirator—annual training.

- *Hazardous electrical voltage safety:* Employees who work with or in the proximity of electrical equipment or systems over 600 V, and are therefore considered a qualified electrical worker—annual training.

Additionally, a continuing education program can benefit an employer while facilitating an employee's knowledge of safe trade practices and requirements. A company can offer monthly or quarterly education courses on specific topics such as working with energized parts, switchboard installations, working on or near power lines, or voltage rating and testing. If you coordinate these trainings with your state or local licensing bureau, these courses may qualify as credit toward an employee getting his/her apprenticeship or journeyman's license. In some cases, companies will offer to compensate employees who choose to take educational courses from outside services or institutions after the worker has successfully completed a class or training module. Voluntary participation or enrollment in education curriculum can be used as a consideration during an employee's performance review. This encourages personnel to expand their skills and knowledge and increase safe workplace practices.

Emergency response plan

OSHA requires employers to have a site-specific employee emergency response plan. This means that all employees must be aware that a clear evacuation plan exists in case of an emergency. Additionally, a risk management plan is required by the EPA if your workplace stores, uses, or will be working around highly hazardous chemicals and materials. Many electrical contractors are not aware that obsolete batteries fall under the category of chemical risks or that installations in a hospital where employees could be exposed to blood qualifies as a hazardous material.

Emergency preparedness means what the name implies—being prepared for emergencies. The goal is to reduce employee injury and property damage in case of an emergency. Situations to consider would be a building collapse, material explosion, or scenarios caused by a natural disaster such as an earthquake or tornado.

Generally, a written emergency plan should contain the following minimum elements:

1. Emergency escape procedures and emergency escape route assignments, based on each job site location.

2. Procedures to account for all employees after emergency evacuation has been completed. This is a pre-established site location where employees must gather in the event of an emergency and includes a method to take attendance and verify that all employees working on the job are present and safe.

3. Rescue and medical duties, if any, for employees who are to perform them.

4. The preferred means for reporting fires and other emergencies.

5. Names or regular job titles of persons or departments to be contacted for further information or explanation of duties under the plan, or to report to in the event of an evacuation or site emergency.

To make the program effective, the emergency action plan should address all potential emergencies that can be expected in the workplace, including civil unrest, tornados, hurricanes, floods, trench or site cave-ins, and other similar emergencies. It's important to consider what emergencies may arise so you can prepare for them before they occur.

What are the emergency action and first aid procedures? The employer should list in detail the procedures to be taken by any employees who may be designated to remain behind to care for essential equipment or operations until their evacuation becomes absolutely necessary, or who are responsible for implementing an emergency plan. Training these personnel is also part of the program. After all, they need information and procedures to put the emergency action plan into action. All employees must be trained in emergency evacuation and the use of floor plans or workplace maps that clearly show routes of evacuation and assembly areas. If you have employees who are hearing impaired or have some type of handicap, your plans must include a specific means of alerting them to an emergency. There are basic training requirements for all employees, so let's take a quick look at some of the training responsibilities:

1. Evacuation plans.

2. Alarm systems and warning horns.

3. Reporting procedures for personnel.

4. Shutdown procedures for equipment and other processes.

5. Types of potential emergencies.

A chain of command should be established to minimize confusion so employees will have no doubt about who has authority for making decisions. Responsible individuals should be identified at the beginning of any project and should have adequate backup so that trained personnel are always available in case of an emergency. During a major emergency involving a fire or explosion, it may be necessary to evacuate site trailers and normal services, such as telephones, electricity, and water may not be available. Planning ahead will help reduce these complications and confusion caused by these problems. There should be a reliable means of communication to handle incoming and outgoing calls, as well as a method of alerting employees to the evacuation location or take other action as required by the situation.

Any warning procedure should be in writing and job foremen need to make sure that every employee knows what signals or alarms mean and what action is to be taken. A method of contacting other personnel including the fire department, police, and hospitals should also be established in advance. Specific employees can be trained as an emergency response team. These people should be trained in emergency procedures, including various types of fire extinguishers and how to properly use them, as well as how to properly shut down electrical power systems. At least one team member should be trained in first aid and CPR. Obviously, the scope of emergency action procedures and written plans depends on the size of the organization and the potential hazards within the workplace. Emergency preparedness saves lives, protects property, and gets you back to work more quickly. There's a lot to emergency planning, and plans should be customized or modified as work locations or site conditions change.

Documentation and record keeping

Numerous record keeping and written program standards are in effect by OSHA, and the best way for a company to prove compliance is to maintain a written, documented paper trail of trainings as well as injuries. There are two major categories of OSHA paperwork compliance: injury and illness record keeping and written programs. Written programs direct the maintenance of many other documents, such as MSDS, which are part of the Hazard Communication Program. There are other incidental paperwork requirements in various OSHA standards that include posting OSHA notices and maintaining inspection records for cranes, chains used in rigging, etc.

Injury and Illness Recordkeeping

The most important records an employer can maintain are logs that document work-related fatalities, injuries, and illnesses. These records are used to compile data on hazardous industries, employers with poor safety performance, and injury and illness trends. OSHA uses the records to help develop and direct its safety compliance assistance, inspection priorities, trade trainings, and intervention strategies.

All electrical contractors with more than 10 employees on the payroll at any point during the year are required to maintain a log of work-related injuries and illnesses, OSHA form 300. This documentation is used to classify injuries and illnesses and their severity. When an incident occurs, the details must be noted in the log, including any injuries or illnesses that result in time lost from work. Other work-related injuries and illnesses that have to be recorded are any events that result in death, loss of consciousness, restricted work activity or temporary job reassignments, or medical treatment that required more than basic first aid. Any accidents that result in a skin-piercing cut from an object that has come in contact with another person's blood or other potentially infectious material also must be recorded. Additionally, cases involving changes in the employee's hearing ability or actual or potential exposure to tuberculosis need to be documented. Companies are required to post a summary of incidents at the end of the year in a visible location so employees are aware of the company's record. The summary needs to be posted annually from February 1 through April 30.

What Qualifies as Work Related?

How do you determine if an injury or illness is truly work related? Well, there are the obvious situations, such as when an employee falls off a ladder, or has debris fall into his eyes while drilling a beam overhead. However, the definition of "work related" is much broader than this. If an event or exposure occurred in the work environment or while an employee was on the clock and it caused or contributed to an employee injury or illness, it is considered work-related. For example, if an employee clocks in at your shop gets his work assignment, loads a company truck and heads to your job site, and ends up injured in an accident on the way, it is considered work-related. He was on the clock, performing one of his required duties, which was driving materials to a job, and he was injured. This is one example of why many employers do not provide their employees with company vehicles that they take home at night. An employee should only be operating a company vehicle as part of performing his job. If he is involved in an accident on the way to the local convenience store while driving a company truck, other people involved in the accident can sue the company rather than the employee. Employees in these circumstances have claimed, and received, workers' compensation because they were injured while operating what is considered company equipment. If the motor vehicle accident occurs on a public street or highway and does not occur in a construction work zone, you do not have to report the incident to OSHA. However, these injuries have to be recorded on your OSHA injury and illness records.

PREEXISTING CONDITIONS

Even preexisting conditions can classify as a work-related injury against your company. How? Well, maybe it will make sense after I tell you Ed's story.

I was the human resource administrator for an area electrical contractor and my boss hired a man named Ed who was a master electrician. Ed had 20 years of experience, so you know right off the bat that he was about 45 years old. When he filled out his employment application, Ed noted that he had experienced problems with one of his knees at his previous job and had arthroscopic surgery to correct a problem with his soft tissue. Ed assured my boss that now his knees were fine and that he no longer had a condition that would prohibit him from performing the duties required of his new position. After about a year with our company, Ed's knees had started bothering him again and he lost his balance walking to his company truck at the end of a work day. He called the office and said he was sure that he was fine, but I made an appointment for him with the company doctor just to make sure. During his visit he told the doctor that he was getting tingling in his legs and that sometimes they felt a bit numb by the end of the day. Our physician did a complete examination of Ed, which included X-rays of his knees and lower back. The tests determined that Ed had developed degenerative disc disease in his spine, and as a result he was experiencing stress on his knees.

The first thing I did was ask the doctor for an explanation of Ed's back condition. Degenerative disc disease is not really a disease but a term used to describe changes in spinal discs as you age. Spinal discs are soft, compressible discs that separate the interlocking vertebra that make up the spine. Normally, the discs act as shock absorbers for the spine, allowing it to flex, bend, and twist. With degenerative disc disease the discs thin out and bone spurs can form as the spine tries to adjust to the inter-vertebral disc changes. The bottom line was that anyone can get degenerative disc disease as they age, whether they are a librarian or a construction worker, so I could not imagine that such a condition would be considered work-related. Furthermore, Ed did not have a diagnosis that was the result of performing his everyday duties and it was not the result of an accident, such as a trip or fall. I understood that Ed's condition could be a disability, but no way could it be a workers' compensation condition, right? Wrong. This scenario is considered aggravation of a preexisting condition, and Ed was out of work on workers' compensation; consequently, I had to record his incident on the OSHA form 300.

FATALITIES AND HOSPITALIZATIONS

OSHA standard 1904.39(a) requires that within 8 hours after the death of any employee from a work-related incident or the in-patient hospitalization of three or more employees as a result of a work-related incident, you must orally report the incident to your area OSHA office. You can do this by calling the central OSHA toll-free telephone number, 1-800-321-OSHA (1-800-321-6742). If you do not learn of a reportable incident at the time it occurs, you must make the report within 8 hs of the time the incident is reported to you. If the fatality was caused by a heart attack, then you need to contact OSHA so that the area office director can decide whether to investigate the incident. This will depend on the circumstances of the heart attack. To report these kinds of circumstances, you will need to provide the following information:

- The establishment name

- The location of the incident

- The time of the incident

- The number of fatalities or hospitalized employees

- The names of any injured employees

- Your contact administrator and his or her phone number

- A brief description of the incident

Additionally, if a fatality or hospitalization happens within 30 days of an accident or occurrence, then you still have to report the incident to OSHA. You do not have to call OSHA to report a fatality or multiple hospitalization incident that occurs when an employee is on a commercial airplane, train, subway, bus, or other public transportation.

Written Hazard Programs

OSHA also has requirements for employers to document compliance with its standards to certify various actions that have been taken. A written program should include a statement of its purpose, the hazard being analyzed, a description of the controls implemented, and methods to evaluate the effectiveness of the program. The purpose of a hazard program is accident and illness prevention. The hazard analysis is a critical element. Depending on the type of hazard, it includes a record of inspections, monitoring, or other tests to determine and document any level of exposure. The controls utilized can be engineering, administrative, or the use of PPE.

Engineering controls include any types of ventilation or equipment that is used to modify the environment, or chemical substitutions that should be used. Administrative controls are the operating practices and procedures, such as an MSDS log, specialized training, an emergency response plan, and first aid training. If applicable, the use of PPE such as respirators should be outlined in the hazard analysis. The use and implementation of these hazard controls should also be evaluated for frequency and effectiveness regularly. Most companies perform an annual program review.

OSHA requires all electrical contractors to develop an accident prevention program (OSHA 1926.20(b)), emergency action plan (OSHA 1926.35), and hazard communication program (OSHA 1926.59). As with a hazard program, an emergency action plan requires an analysis of possible emergencies that can occur. This plan needs to describe the controls to be used, such as an emergency notification plan, escape procedures, and training. The hazard communication program requires an inspection of the workplace and job sites for hazardous chemicals, to ensure proper labeling of chemicals, an MSDS log to identify the chemical hazards, and procedures for controlling hazardous exposure through training on handling hazards. A respiratory protection program (OSHA 1926.103) is required if there are airborne hazards and should include medical examination and assessment to ensure that employees are capable of wearing the respirators. Equipment fit-test records and procedures for the use and maintenance of respirators should also be documented. If electrical installations or maintenance are performed in a work area where noise levels exceed 85 decibels, then OSHA 1926.52 requires hearing protection to be worn.

Similar written programs are outlined in OSHA 1910.146 for permit-required confined spaces, and OSHA 1910.147 regarding controlling hazardous energy—lockout/tagout.

The National Fire Protection Association (NFPA) 70E Standard for Electrical Safety in the Workplace contains documentation requirements for possible exposures, and implementation of the OSHA programs described above are used to demonstrate compliance.

PRE-JOB SAFETY BRIEFINGS

The purpose of a pre-job safety briefing is to help workers and supervisors establish a clear understanding of the scope of work that will be performed each day and to identify potential hazards that could adversely impact employees, the public, the environment, or the facility/site and its equipment. This goal is achieved by discussing and documenting the tasks that will be involved, potential hazards, and safety precautions that will need to be taken. It provides workers and supervisors the opportunity to clarify the objectives, personnel roles and responsibilities, and resources that are needed to safely perform the day's work. The supervisor should be responsible for understanding the scope of work clearly enough to plan the day's work, identify hazards associated with the work, and to develop necessary schedules, priorities, and safety-based work instructions. The goal here is to ensure the safe performance of work, provide clear guidance on how to apply any safety controls, and still allow enough appropriate flexibility so that employees can accomplish their work without unnecessary restrictions, costs, or burdens.

A pre-job briefing does not need to be long-winded or overly time consuming. One of the best ways to keep a safety briefing short and sweet is to use a standard job safety briefing form. This tool also provides documentation that a pre-job briefing was held (Figure 2.6).

JOB SAFETY ANALYSIS			Date:	
Prepared by:		**Project Name or Number:**	**Site Address:**	
Work Scope/Description:				
Emergency Contact Person:			**Pre-job Walkthrough Conducted:**	☐ Yes ☐ No

PART 1

Hazards Associated with this Job (MEKGO) *Circle All Applicable and Address in PART 2*

Mechanical	**E**lectrical	**K**inetic	**G**ravity	**O**ther
Equipment failure	Electrical contact	Traffic	Falling from a height	Asbestos
Conductor tension	Induced voltage	Driving conditions	Falling objects	Confined space
Cable tension	Back-feed	Moving/shifting loads	Climbing obstructions	Excavations
Moving parts	Flash potential	Rotating machinery	Aerial device operation	Pressurized fluids/gases
Loads-hoisting/rigging	Energized Parts	Heavy equip. operation		Weather Conditions

PRESENT OR POTENTIAL SAFETY HAZARDS

	Yes	No	Reference			Yes	No	Reference
Hot Work Requires a permit/form/report	☐	☐	OSHA 29CFRl926 Subparts F & J	**Scaffolding**	☒ ☑	☐	☐	OSHA 29CRF1926 Subpart L
Lock and Tag Requires a permit/form/report	☒ ☑	☐	☐	OSHA 29CFRl910.47	**Aerial Lifts/ Bucket Work**	☒ ☑	☐	☐	OSHA 29CRF1926 Subpart N
Fall Hazards (>6 ft)	☒ ☑	☐	☐	OSHA 29CRF1926 Subpart M	**Hazardous Materials**	☒	☐	☐	OSHA 29CRF1926.59
Noise	☒	☐	☐	OSHA 29CFRl910.95	**Excavation/Trenching** Requires a permit/form/report	☑	☐	☐	OSHA 29CRF1926 Subpart P
Confined Space Requires a permit/form/report	☒ ☑	☐	☐	OSHA 29CRF1910 Subpart J	**Site/Vehicle Traffic**		☐	☐	See Company Policy

☑ = Requires certification or competent/qualified person designation   ☒ = Requires formal/special training

MINIMUM DRESS/PPE REQUIREMENTS:

Have all required permits, forms or reports been completed and filed?	☐ Yes	☐ No

PART 2

DESCRIBE PLANNED ACTIVITIES AND ANY ASSOCIATED HAZARDS	SAFE WORK CONTROLS

Figure 2.6   Using a standardized pre-job safety briefing form keeps meetings effective and efficient.

Ultimately, the effectiveness of a pre-job briefing depends on advanced preparation and assessment of the work conditions by a supervisor. This means the job foreman can't show up 5 min before the shift starts and have a clear understanding of hazards present for the days's work. Planning the work is an essential part of any safety management program, and the supervisor should ask workers if they know of any existing risks or safety issues. Many companies use a graded approach, such as a scale of 1-10, to categorize a job's potential hazards and complexity.

The job assessment should include daily site conditions such as weather, mud, need for snow removal, icy conditions, and the like. Basic safety compliance standards should be in place, such as the use of ground fault circuit interrupters (GFCIs) on all extension cords and portable power tools, an equipment check, and verification that all workers are wearing applicable PPE. A site safety checklist can provide a concise assessment of typical electrical requirements, such as:

- Visually inspect electrical equipment before use. Take any defective equipment out of service.

- Ground all power supply systems, electrical circuits, and electrical equipment.

- Inspect electrical systems to ensure that the path to ground is continuous.

- Confirm that ground prongs from cord- and plug-connected equipment or extension cords have not be removed.

- Make sure that double-insulated tools are onsite.

- Ground all exposed metal parts of equipment.

- Avoid standing in wet areas when using portable electrical equipment.

If a specific safety issue exists, such as the use of generators on site, the foreman should provide more specific direction for safe work practices (Figures 2.7–2.9).

The supervisor should also take time to complete any supplemental hazard assessment documentation, such as confined space permits or energized work permits, prior to conducting a pre-job briefing.

GENERATORS

Most generators are gasoline powered and use internal combustion engines to produce electricity. They produce Carbon monoxide, which, when inhaled, reduces your ability to utilize oxygen.

Symptoms of carbon monoxide poisoning include headache, nausea and tiredness that can lead to unconsciousness and ultimately prove fatal.

SAFETY CONTROLS:

✗ DO NOT bring a generator indoors. Be sure it is located outdoors in a location where the exhaust gases cannot enter a home or building.

✗ Be sure that the main circuit breaker is OFF and locked out prior to starting any generator. This will prevent inadvertent energization of power lines from back feed electrical energy from generators.

✗ Turn off generators and let them cool prior to refueling.

Figure 2.7 Pre-printed handouts can be provided for typical safe work practice scenarios.

EXTENSION CORDS

Normal wear on cords can loosen or expose wires. Cords that are not 3-wire type, not designed for hard-usage, or that have been modified, increase the risk of contacting electrical current.

SAFETY CONTROLS:

✗ Use only equipment that is approved to meet OSHA standards.

✗ Do not modify cords or use them incorrectly.

✗ Use factory-assembled cord sets and only extension cords that are 3-wire type.

✗ Use only cords, connection devices, and fittings that are equipped with strain relief.

✗ Remove cords from receptacles by pulling on the plugs, not the cords..

Figure 2.8 Check extension cords to insure they are in safe operational condition.

POWER LINES

Overhead and buried power lines are especially hazardous because they carry extremely high voltage. Fatal electrocution is the main risk, but burns and falls are also hazards.

SAFETY CONTROLS:

- Look for overhead power lines. Stay at least 10 feet away from overhead power lines and assume they are energized.
- Locate buried power lines in advance by contacting a Dig-Safe firm to make power line locations.
- De-energize and ground lines when working near them.
- Use non-conductive wood or fiberglass ladders when working near power lines.

Figure 2.9   Ensure safe conditions when working near power lines.

Reliance versus compliance

On-going safety trainings are proven to help reduce the incidence of work place injuries. The key to any safety program's success is for employees to become reliant on safety protocols and see them as a priority. Most employees will grudgingly observe the major points of their employer's safety requirements when they know that compliance is mandatory. However, when employees believe in the value and importance of safe work practices they will strive to incorporate safety into their workday. They will become safety-conscious because they are informed and educated and they understand that their safety and the safety of their co-workers is important to their employer and to their own well-being. Safety-focused employees should be encouraged, acknowledged, and rewarded for their efforts. You can consider awarding them with anything from a certificate of appreciation, to a free lunch, to earned comp time. This type of recognition can inspire other employees to increase their safety efforts. In the end, you will have developed a workforce that willingly seeks to make safety a priority in each workday. The result will be reductions in injuries, lost time, citations, overhead, and job delays. Everyone will be able to go home at the end of the day in the same shape they were in when they reported for work, and everyone will benefit (Figure 2.00).

Elements of a Electrical Safety Manual

Section 1 — Management and Employee Involvement

- Statements on the value of workplace safety and management's committed to safety
- List of company contacts, such as the name and phone extension of the Safety Director
- Statement that adherence to all safety and health rules is a condition of employment

Section 2 — Hazard Prevention and Control

- Process for employee safety, tool, PPE, and equipment training and mandatory participation
- List of safety expectations, such as:

  - Employees will wear PPE appropriate for the work to be performed
  - Employees will examine cords and equipment for damage prior to use, and will report any damaged items and remove them from use
  - Employees will report any site hazards to the job supervisor immediately
  - Employees will report any work-related injuries to their supervisor or Safety Director within 24 hours
  - Requirements for use of company vehicles and reporting vehicular accidents

- List of unacceptable employee actions and consequences, such as:

  - Drug or alcohol use
  - Horseplay
  - Harassment of other employees or clients
  - Smoking, other than in areas designated for smoking
  - Ramifications of violating safety protocols, including verbal warnings and suspensions

- List of emergency procedures
- Accident reporting and investigation procedures

Element 3 — Safety and Health Education

- Policy to allow only properly authorized and trained employees to perform specific work
- Provision to hold emergency-preparedness drills using a range of scenarios for employees
- Method for training supervisors and managers to recognize hazards and understand their responsibilities
- Location of MSDS on each job site
- Provision for first aid, CPR, and other health and safety trainings
- Policies regarding Workers Compensation, Return To Work, and Re-training programs

Figure 2.00 Key elements for a comprehensive Safety Manual.

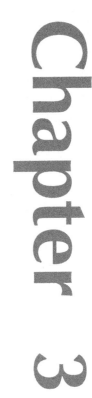

Chapter 3

Recognizing the Real Dangers of Electricity

▌ What is electricity?

Electricity is the energy formed by the imbalanced movement of electrons and protons. This movement creates an electrical charge, and just like the flow of a river, electrical flow is referred to as electrical

45

current. Electric current has three effects: heat, chemical, and magnetic. The most common electrical hazard we encounter on a regular basis is from heat (Figure 3.1).

In our daily lives we use a variety of devices that convert electrical energy into heat energy, light energy, chemical energy, or mechanical energy. Let's start with a quick science lesson to gain an understanding of the characteristics of electricity. When electric current is passed through a metallic wire, like the filaments of an electric heater or oven, the filament gets heated up. This is known as the heating effect of current. This heat is generated because a metallic conductor has a large number of free electrons in it. When a potential difference is applied across the ends of a metallic wire, the free electrons begin to drift from the low potential to the high potential region. This allows the electrons to collide with the positive ions, or protons, and the collisions release the energy in electrons. Since positive ions are atoms that do not have any electrons, the collisions transfer the electron energy to the protons and they begin to vibrate violently. As a result, heat is produced. The greater the number of electrons flowing per second, the larger the collision rate and the more heat will be produced. When the human body or any combustible material comes in contact with this process, burning can result.

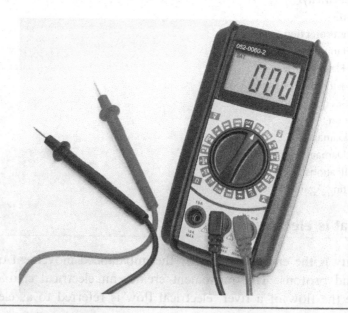

Figure 3.1   The presence of electrical current can be tested using an amp or a volt meter.

Fire hazards

Combustible materials include paper, wood, and clothing, as well as fine particles such as flour, saw dust, and coal dust. Additionally, gases and fuels, such as gasoline, are highly combustible. For this reason, a variety of job sites and working conditions pose potential fire hazards that can be ignited when they come in contact with electrical current. The National Fire Protection Association (NFPA) publishes codes relating to fire, electrical hazard, and building safety. OSHA requested that the NFPA develop a specific standard addressing electrical safe work practices. In response, the first edition of NFPA 70E was published. Both OSHA and NFPA have a number of regulations relating to protecting workers and property from fire damage.

Always use the correct size fuse. Replacing a fuse with one of a larger size can cause excessive currents in the wiring and possibly start a fire.

OSHA fire protection standards

OSHA Section 1926.151 defines ignition hazards for construction sites. It requires electrical wiring and equipment for light, heat, or power purposes to be installed in compliance with the requirements of OSHA Subpart K for electrical work. By the way, this section also prohibits smoking at or in the vicinity of operations that could constitute a fire hazard, and for these areas to be posted: "No Smoking or Open Flame." These areas could include trash or lumber piles, areas where gas heaters are used, or areas near propane tanks, gas cans, or even paint cans.

Any portable battery powered lighting equipment that will be used in connection with the storage, handling, or use of flammable gases or liquids has to be approved for hazardous locations. Additionally, bonding devices cannot be attached or detached in areas with hazardous concentrations of flammable gases or vapors.

Portable fire extinguishing equipment that is not rated any less than 2A that is suitable for any potential fire hazard has to be provided at convenient, conspicuously accessible locations on the construction site.

"Accessible" means that extinguishers are located at a maximum distance of 100 feet to the nearest work location.

Construction materials, including piles of conduit or coils of wire have to be stored in a way that does not obstruct, or adversely affect, any exits from buildings. A clearance of 24 inches has to be maintained around the path of travel of fire doors and no materials can be stored or piled within 36 inches of a fire door opening. Additionally, you have to allow a clearance of at least 36 inches between the top level of any stored material and any sprinkler deflectors. OSHA also requires that you allow clearance around lights and any heating units to prevent ignition of combustible materials (Figure 3.2).

While we are talking about clearances, OSHA even has regulations for using salamander and other portable heaters. For those of us who work in Maine, these heaters are commonplace on construction sites. According to OSHA, these heaters have to be suitable for use on wood floors if you plan on setting them up on plywood or any other combustible material. Otherwise, you have to set them on a suitable heat insulating material or they have to be on at least 1 inch of concrete.

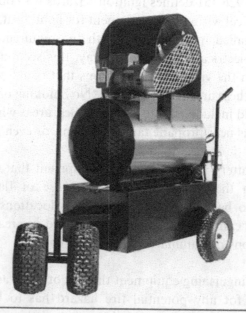

Figure 3.2   Space heaters must be kept away from all flammable materials.

The insulating material has to extend beyond the heater 2 feet or more in all directions. Also, be sure to clear the area around these heaters 10 feet in all directions from any tarpaulins, canvas, or plastic sheeting. Before you start up a portable heater make sure any tarps or coverings are securely fastened to prevent ignition or upsetting of the heater if the wind starts moving the covering around.

Containers of solvent, conduit glue, or any other flammable or combustible liquids cannot be left in areas used for exits or stairways. Finally, any materials that could react with water and create a fire hazard cannot be stored in the same room with flammable or combustible liquids.

If you are working in damp locations, inspect electric cords and equipment to ensure that they are in good condition and free of defects, and use a ground-fault circuit interrupter to prevent electrical shock.

NEC FLAMMABLE CONDITIONS

The National Electrical Code addresses in Chapter 5 hazardous conditions that create the potential for fires to occur. Environments that pose fire or combustion hazards are listed in Articles 500-510. Requirements covering specific types of facilities that pose additional hazards, such as bulk storage plants or motor fuel dispensing locations, are explained in Articles 511-516.

NEC Section (C)(2)(1) describes Class II, Division 2 locations classifications. These are listed as:

1. Locations where some combustible dust is normally in the air but where abnormal operations may increase the suspended dust to ignitable or explosive levels.

2. Locations where combustible dust accumulations are normally not concentrated enough to interfere with the operation of electrical equipment unless an "infrequent equipment malfunction" occurs that increases the level of dust suspended in the air.

3. Locations where combustible dust concentrations in or on electrical equipment may be sufficient to limit heat dissipation or that could be ignited by failure or abnormal operation of electrical equipment.

A variety of airborne environmental conditions that require classification are listed in Article 500. Class I covers locations specified in Sections [500.5(B)(1)] and [500.5 (B)(2)] where flammable gases or vapors are present, or could exist in the air in high enough quantities that they could produce explosive or ignitable mixtures. Section [500.5(B)(1) FPN 1] provides examples of locations usually included in Class I as the following:

1. Where volatile flammable liquids or liquefied flammable gases are transferred from one container to another.

2. Interiors of spray booths and areas in the vicinity of spraying and painting operations where volatile flammable solvents are used.

3. Locations containing open tanks or vats of volatile flammable liquids.

4. Drying rooms or compartments for the evaporation of flammable solvents.

5. Locations with fat and oil extraction equipment that uses volatile flammable solvents.

6. Portions of cleaning and dyeing plants where flammable liquids are used.

7. Gas generator rooms and other portions of gas manufacturing plants where flammable gas may escape.

8. Pump rooms for flammable gas or for volatile flammable liquids that are not adequately ventilated.

9. The interiors of refrigerators and freezers where flammable materials are stored in open or easily ruptured containers.

10. All other locations where ignitable concentrations of flammable vapors or gases are likely to occur in the course of normal operations.

Class I lists group *air mixtures* that are not oxygen-enriched. These include the following:

■ Group A—Acetylene.

■ Group B—Flammable gas, flammable vapors which produce liquid, and combustible vapor mixed with air that could burn or explode with a maximum experimental safe gap (MESG) value *equal to or less than 0.45 mm* or with a minimum igniting current ratio (MIC ratio) *equal to or less than 0.04.*

■ Group C—Flammable gas, flammable vapors which produce liquid, and combustible vapor mixed with air that could burn or explode with an MESG value *greater than 0.45 mm* but less than 0.75 mm or an MIC ratio *greater than 0.04* but less than 0.80.

■ Group D—Flammable gas, flammable vapors which produce liquid, and combustible vapor mixed with air that could burn or explode with an MESG value *greater than 0.75* or a MIC ratio *greater than 0.80* (Figure 3.3).

Class II locations continue the group classifications for environments affected by *combustible dusts,* as follows:

■ Group E—Atmospheres containing combustible metal dusts whose particle abrasiveness, size, or conductivity pose hazards in the use of electrical equipment.

■ Group F—Atmospheres containing combustible carbonaceous dusts, such as coal and charcoal, which present an explosion hazard.

■ Group G—Atmospheres containing combustible dusts that are not already included in Group E or F, such as wood or plastic dust, grain, or chemical dust.

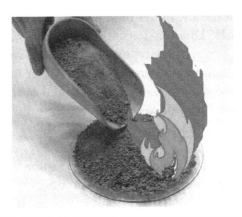

Figure 3.3 Combustible dust is made of fine particles that are easily ignited.

The approved protection techniques for these group locations are found in NEC Section [500.7].

Article 501 states that a Class I hazardous (classified) location is an area where flammable gases or vapors may be present in quantities sufficient to produce an explosive or ignitable mixture. Article 501 contains installation requirements for these locations, including wiring methods, equipment connections, and devices. Equipment installations that are included under this classification are:

- General power distribution

- Transformers and capacitors—Section [501.2]

- Meters, instruments and relays—Section [501.3]

- Wiring methods—Section [501.4]

- Seals and drainage requirements—Section [501.5]

- Controls, such as covers switches, fuses, circuit breakers, or motor controllers—Section [501.6]

- Transformers and resistors—Section [501.7]

- Motors and generators, load requirements, luminaires, flexible cords, receptacles, and conductor insulation—Sections [501.8-501.13]

- Surge protection in these hazardous areas—Section [501.17]

Article 502 specifically addresses conditions and locations that contain combustible dust in the air, rather than just the presence of combustible materials. A Class II, Division 1 location is one in which combustible dust is present in the air under normal operating conditions in high enough quantities that it could produce explosive or ignitable mixtures. Additionally, if a mechanical failure or abnormal operation of machinery or equipment might produce combustible dust, then those locations or facilities would fall under Class II, Division I.

A Class II, Division 2 location is defined as a location where combustible dust is present in large enough quantities to produce explosive or ignitable mixtures due to the abnormal operation of systems. If combustible dust accumulations are present but are normally insufficient to interfere with the normal operation of electrical equipment, unless an infrequent equipment malfunction occurred, then this situation is covered under Class II, Division 2 as well. Finally, combustible dust accumulations on, in, or in the vicinity of the electrical equipment that could interfere with the safe dissipation of heat from electrical equipment, or which could be ignited by an electrical equipment failure, are also included in this section.

Article 503 lists Class III locations as areas where fibers or filings could be easily ignited. The classification standard that separates these locations from the previous ones is that if you don't have enough fibers in the air to produce an ignitable mixture but they are present, then it is a Class III area. Typical examples of a Class III location would be a textile or saw mill or a clothing manufacturing plant. Class III, Division 2 locations are similar except that these are locations where ignitable fibers are stored or handled.

The reason you need to be aware of all these conditions it so you can be proactive in preventing fires that could result from sparks, live wires, the use of strikers or torches, or any other conditions that could arise during the course of electrical installations or repairs.

Blast and flash injuries

Electricity can cause two types of burns: electrical burns from direct contact with current and thermal burns from arc flashes and blasts. It's expected that the explosive energy released during an arc blast will send more than 2000 North American electrical workers to burn centers each year. Injuries caused by an electrical arc include concussion, burns, and impalement. So what causes an arc flash and arc blast? A short-circuit or fault occurs when the insulation between energized electrical phase conductors, or between a phase conductor and ground, is damaged, absent, or compromised. During a "bolted" fault, the fault current flows over a conductive path, but only a little energy is released into the surrounding environment during the fault. During an arcing fault, however, the fault current flows through the air rather than through a conductor or busbar and a great deal of thermal energy is released into the environment. This sudden release of thermal energy is referred to as an arc-flash event.

An arc flash occurs when powerful, high-amperage currents travel, or arc, through the air. This can occur when high voltage differences exist across a gap between conductors. The result is an instant release of tremendous amounts of energy. Temperatures as high as 36,000°F have been recorded in arc flashes.

The arc fault current is less than the available bolted fault current and below the rating of circuit breakers, which means these will not trip and the full force of an arc flash will occur. The electrical equation for energy is volts X current X time. The transition from arc fault to arc flash increases in intensity as the pressure wave develops.

Factors that can contribute to an arc flash or blast include:

1. The available short circuit current.

2. Dirt buildup in the equipment that may affect the conductive path.

3. Moisture and humidity.

4. Circuit supply voltage.

5. Continuous motor operation during a fault.

Hazards From an Arc Flash or Blast

The intense heat and light emitted by an arc flash can cause severe burns, destroying skin and tissue. An arc flash can ignite or melt clothing, resulting in further burns. Blast victims often require skin grafts and sometimes even amputations. A high-amperage arc can produce a pressure wave blast with a force of up to 3000 pounds per square foot. The victim can be thrown by the force of this pressure, resulting in concussion injuries or impalement from flying metal. Injuries can occur from falling or colliding with nearby objects. Hearing loss may also result from damaging sound levels and excessive pressure. Pressure waves in excess of 720 lbs/ft^2 can rupture eardrums, and between 1728 to 2160 lbs/ft^2 pressures can cause lungs to collapse (Figure 3.4).

The intense heat may melt metal electrical components and blast molten droplets considerable distances. These droplets harden rapidly and can

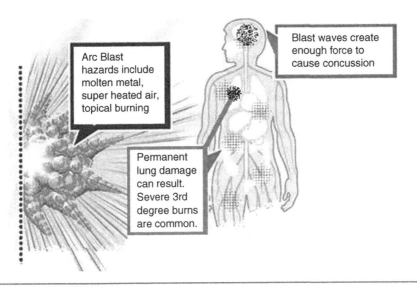

Arc Blast hazards include molten metal, super heated air, topical burning

Blast waves create enough force to cause concussion

Permanent lung damage can result. Severe 3rd degree burns are common.

Figure 3.4   Super-heated air, molten metal particles and fire injuries are common in an arc blast.

lodge in a person's skin, ignite clothing, and may cause lung damage. Just imagine the effects of breathing in hot, molten metal laden air. As severe as these injuries can be, the most severe result of an arc blast is death. The incidence of death is more likely with increased severity of burns, the percent of body area affected, and age (Figure 3.5).

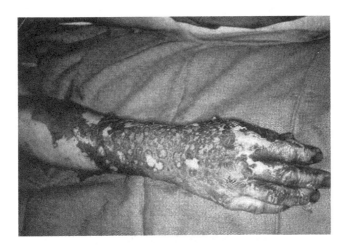

Figure 3.5   Without using proper precautions and PPE, severe burns can result from an arc flash.

OSHA Requirements

OSHA 1910.303 requires employers to mark electrical equipment with descriptive markings, including the equipment's voltage, current, wattage, or other ratings as necessary. OSHA believes that this information, along with the training requirements for qualified persons, will provide employees the necessary information to protect themselves from arc-flash hazards.

Additionally, in 1910.335(b), OSHA requires employers to use alerting techniques, such as safety signs and tags, barricades, and attendants to warn and protect workers from hazards that could cause electric shock, burns, or failure of electric equipment parts. Although OSHA Subpart S electrical provisions do not specifically require that electric equipment has to be marked to identify potential arc-flash hazards, OSHA 1910.335(b)(1) requires the use of safety signs and symbols to warn employees about electrical hazards, including electric-arc-flash hazards, which could endanger them under the general terms of OSHA 1910.145. This OSAH section requires the use of signs or symbols to indicate or define specific hazards that could lead to accidental injury to workers or the public, or to property damage (Figure 3.6).

Compliance with OSHA requires an employer to adhere to several key points, including:

- Provide and be able to demonstrate a safety program with defined responsibilities, including training for workers on the hazards of arc flash.

- Ensure that "appropriate" personal protective equipment (PPE) is worn by workers.

- The employer must require workers to use appropriate tools.

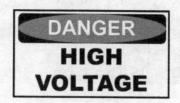

Figure 3.6   OSHA requires certain equipment to be labeled with warning signs.

- Warning labels must be affixed to equipment. This is the responsibility of the equipment owners, not the manufacturers. Warning labels should include the equipment's flash protection boundary, its incident energy level, and the required PPE.

- Prior to working on any energized equipment, a qualified person must perform calculations to assess the degree of potential arc flash hazard.

The term "appropriate" was vague and fairly ambiguous for a long time, and it left the door open for employers to say that in their opinion they had provided adequate protection for their employees against electrical hazards. This problem was solved when NFPA published Section 70E, which specifically addresses electrical safety and the means required to determine what constitutes "appropriate" precautions. NFPA 70E contains hazard calculation methods, examples, and PPE charts to aid employers in taking effective, appropriate safety precautions.

Electrocution

"If you haven't been hit at least once, then you're not ready to hold an electrician's license." I heard a master electrician say that to a helper one day; the "hit" he was referring to was a jolt of electricity. This statement, and other similar comments, demonstrates the misplaced idea that electricity is no big deal and that everyone who works with electricity should expect and accept some level of contact with a live circuit. I know electricians who tell stories of testing wires by licking their fingers then touching the conductor. These workers are accidents waiting to happen.

Always use ladders made of wood or other non-conductive materials when working with or near electricity.

It has been estimated that at least 700 occupational electrocutions occur in the U.S. each year, but this figure is based only on reported accidents. The National Electrical Code divides voltages into two categories: greater than 600 V (high voltage) and less than or equal to 600 V (low voltage).

BRAIN DAMAGE

In the same way that electricity travels through a wire, current can flow through your body by moving across or through blood vessels, nerves, muscles, and cells. In more serious electrocution accidents, electrons flowing abnormally through your body can produce injury or death by depolarizing (tearing apart) muscles and nerves, initiating abnormal electrical rhythms in the heart and brain, or producing internal and external electrical burns. Burns can be the result of heating or from current boring thermal holes in cell membranes. Just think of it as if someone was firing a microscopic laser through your body. Current passing through the brain, in both low-voltage and high-voltage circuits, often produces unconsciousness instantly because of the depolarization of the brain's neurons. This is not because blood flow is suddenly restricted to the brain. It is because the nerve impulses in the brain have been disrupted. In this example, think of your brain like a computer that is not plugged into a surge protector when lightning strikes. Your hard drive could get completely fried, or at a bare minimum incredibly fragmented. It is harder to defrag your brain than it is your computer. There is another risk of brain damage from an electrical shock that results if you stop breathing. Circuits that pass through a person for a matter of minutes produce ischemic* brain damage if they interfere with respiratory movement.

*Definition: Ischemic is the damage caused by a decreased flow of oxygenated blood to any part of the body.

High and low voltage circuits can produce myonecrosis (death of individual muscle fibers), and myoglobinemia (the rapid breakdown of skeletal muscle tissue proteins), and the complications that come with these conditions (Figure 3.7).

HEART DAMAGE

Now let's talk about your heart. Not your sensitive side, but that other vital organ that has to work just right to keep you alive. Even though brief contact with low voltages seldom produces a thermal or burn injury, it can still cause a very rapid, ineffective heartbeat,

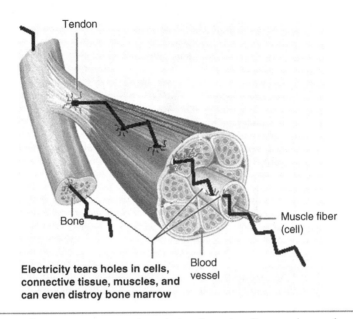

Tendon

Bone

Muscle fiber
(cell)

Electricity tears holes in cells, Blood
connective tissue, muscles, and vessel
can even distroy bone marrow

Figure 3.7 Electricity can tear or burn holes through cells, muscles, and connective tissue.

known as ventricular fibrillation. So to any electricians out there who don't think a "hit" is anything to worry about, just remember that your heart is designed to beat with a regular rhythm, not an ineffective one. Alternating current (AC) can produce ventricular fibrillation if the path of the current involves a passage through the chest. This can happen when the current flows from arm-to-arm, arm-to-leg, or from your head to your arm or leg. In situations involving contact with high voltage, massive current flows can stop the heart completely. When contact to the electrical supply is broken, the heart may start beating normally, or it may not. Forced respiration by immediate mouth-to-mouth techniques may be required, even if a heartbeat and pulse are present, to ensure that the heart re-establishes a normal rhythm. Anytime you have two contact points, one with a source of energy and the other with a source of ground, you are almost guaranteed that electricity is going to pass through your heart. Your heart is a muscle, which means that it is susceptible to tissue damage and it relies on electrical signals from your brain to beat normally. That means that your risk of permanent physical damage is very high when external current passes through your heart (Figure 3.8).

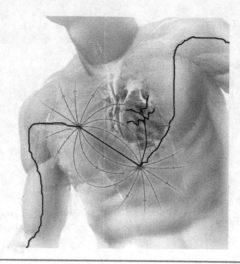

Figure 3.8 Electrical current passing through your heart is similar to the shock of a defibrillator used to resuscitate heart attack victims in an emergency room.

Electrocution victims can be revived if immediate cardiopulmonary resuscitation (CPR) or defibrillation is provided. While immediate defibrillation would be ideal, CPR given within approximately 4 minutes of the electrocution, followed by advanced cardiac life support (ACLS) measures within approximately 8 minutes, can be lifesaving.

COMPLICATIONS FROM ELECTROCUTION

We have already established that electrical current can produce burns with relatively massive amounts of skin and tissue destruction. This type of injury results from joule heating which is the term used for the friction created by rapidly moving electrons. Thermal burns that result from electrocution are considered complications or secondary injuries caused by the electrocution. That is, unless the burns are so extensive that death results from subsequent complications. Additional complications from electrocution include nerve, organ, and soft tissue damage. Remember that old song about the parts of the body that connect to each other? Well, in the case of electrocution, the destruction caused by electrical current coursing through the body can have delayed and lingering effects to parts of the body that you would not even think about. For example, your sense of taste or smell can be diminished, your vision can be affected, and you can lose feeling in your extremities. Some of the damage that you might not think about can be to organs such as your stomach or bladder as a result of spasms caused by an electrical current. Other organs that rely on small components to function properly, such as the bronchioles in your lungs or the cilia in your intestines can be temporarily or permanently damaged (Figure 3.9).

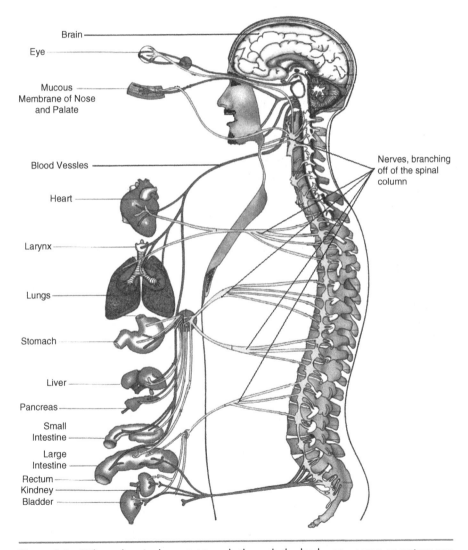

Figure 3.9 When electrical current travels through the body, any organ or system can be damaged.

PROTECTING AGAINST ELECTRICAL CURRENT

Anyone can be exposed to the dangers of electricity while at work, from lose or frayed cords to defective equipment, but by the very nature of their jobs electricians have an increased chance of injury. Most electrical accidents occur because individuals are working on or near equipment that was thought to be dead but which is not, or they are working on or near equipment which they know is live, but they think they have enough experience so they don't take adequate precautions.

> Know where the breakers and boxes are located on your worksite so that you can cut the power in case of an emergency.

Sometimes it is something as simple as misusing equipment or using equipment that is faulty. Because electricity can be so damaging to workers, employers, employees and self-employed electricians need to take precautions to make sure that electrical systems are constructed and installed in a way that prevents danger and only work on, use, or de-energize electrical systems in a way that prevents danger. Additionally, all workers should be conscious of potential electrical hazards from damaged cords, power tools and equipment, and combustible debris. Tools should always be turned off before they are unplugged and no one should ever pull an extension cord out of an outlet by tugging on the cord. Tools and power equipment, such as generators, need to be turned off before anyone makes any adjustments to them or adds fuel.

If an injury does occur you are obliged to report incidents that involve injury from an electric shock or electrical burn that result in unconsciousness or require resuscitation or admittance to a hospital. You must also report injuries from an electrical short circuit or overload that causes a fire or explosion or involves contact with overhead power lines.

The most important thing to remember is that everyone who works with electricity needs to be responsible for assessing, implementing, and promoting safeguards against injuries caused by electrical current (Figure 3.00).

EFFECTS OF ELECTRICAL SHOCK

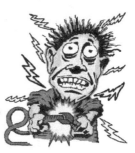

Electric shock is the physical stimulation that occurs when electric current flows through the human body. The distribution of current flow through the body depends on the resistance of the various paths that the current flows through. The final trauma associated with the electric shock is determined by the most critical path called the Shock Circuit.

Burns: caused by electric current occur from the inside of the body. Electric current burns typically impact vital internal organs, destroying tissue and growth centers. External damage to skin results in third-degree burns, blistering and scarring.

Cell Wall Damage; cell death can result from the enlargement of cellular pores due to high-intensity electrical pulse through the cells, known as "electroporation". This process allows ions to flow freely through the cell membranes, causing cell death.

Current Flow: Electrical shock current flow tends to follow the same current paths used by the body's central nervous system. Since the external current is much higher than the body's normal current flow, damage is done to the nervous system, including deterioration of destruction of the myelin sheath which covers and protects nerves.

Damage- Nervous System: Electrical current destroys neurons, melanon, and nerve synapses. Since the nervous system is the communications pathway used to control the muscles, nerve damage can result in loss of senses such as touch, smell and taste, or muscle function.

Damage – Muscles: Currents as low as 5 amps will cause muscle and tissue damage. Electrical current results in deep muscle damage which may not present as a complication for days or months until the muscle tissue begins to shrink or atrophy. The heart is a muscle and, like any muscle, it can become paralyzed and damaged if external current flows through it.

Electric Hold: The reaction of muscles to uncontrollably contract when an electric current passes through them. Your muscles clench to anything you are holding or touching and you cannot let go. Consequently, the electric shock will continue until the current is cut-off or another person intervenes and physically frees you from the contact with the current. The flow of current through tissue causes heating which will make the body's resistance drop, resulting in an increase in the current.

Fibrillation: This is the rapid and inefficient contraction of muscle fibers of the heart caused by disruption of nerve impulses. If the heart can not regain normal rhythm quickly, it will stop beating altogether.

Figure 3.00   Electrical shock effects the body in a variety of damaging ways.

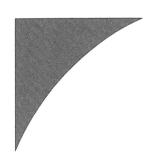

Working on Energized Parts and Equipment

Chapter 4

Chapter Outline

It has been said that "knowledge is power." When working with electrical power, knowledge is the difference between who can work on energized systems and who cannot. Employees are segregated into several categories: qualified, competent, unqualified, and non-essential

65

Doi: 10.1016/B978-1-85617-654-5.00004-2

personnel. A few years of experience in the electrical trade do not automatically equate to you being considered competent or a qualified worker. Here are the factors that do determine your level of service.

Qualified workers

An electrician can be qualified to complete certain electrical tasks, but not qualified to complete others. This means that the fundamental factor that determines your status as a qualified electrician depends on the work to be performed. The determining factors are technical expertise and knowledge of the electrical safe work practices necessary for the task at hand. One exception would be an apprentice or other worker who is undergoing training to become a qualified person. These employees are actually considered qualified if they are under the direct supervision of a qualified person.

Expertise is a quality that must be demonstrated or documented. One method of proving expertise is through specific training or certifications. OSHA 29 CFR 1926.32(l) considers a person "qualified" if they possess a recognized degree or certificate. Numerous colleges throughout the U.S. offer degree programs for electricians. Typical curriculums for electrician degree programs include the following:

- National Electrical Code
- Electrical blueprint reading
- Fundamentals of electricity
- Electrical safety
- Electrical wiring
- Technical math
- Introduction to mechanics
- Electrical circuits
- Industrial wiring
- Technical writing

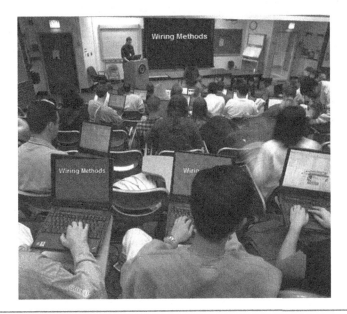

Figure 4.1 Many colleges and vocational programs offer degree courses for electricians.

- Electric zone heating

- Residential wiring

- Motor control diagrams

- Solid state devices

- Occupational math

Many experienced tradesmen believe that no amount of book learning can compare with hands-on experience. However, even seasoned electricians are often required to increase their academic understanding of the trade. This is why many states require continuing education courses as a requisite to renewing a master electrician license. Such stipulations encourage tradesmen to broaden their fact-based knowledge, beyond basic hands-on experience. Typical certification courses include practical topics such as National Electrical Code changes, temporary wiring installations, energized systems, grounding and bonding safety, electrical theory and application, and modules that focus on alternating current, motors, generators, or transformers.

The OSHA Training Institute (OTI) provides training and education in occupational safety and health for the private sector. Contact your state OSHA office for details.

Electricians often complete regular safety programs, manufacturer-specific training, and management training courses that provide the tradesman with certification. Joint training committees made up of local unions of the International Brotherhood of Electrical Workers and local chapters of the National Electrical Contractors Association, individual electrical contracting companies, or local chapters of the Associated Builders and Contractors and the Independent Electrical Contractors Association often sponsor certified training programs as well. Even OSHA sponsors an accredited 30-hour construction course (Figure 4.2).

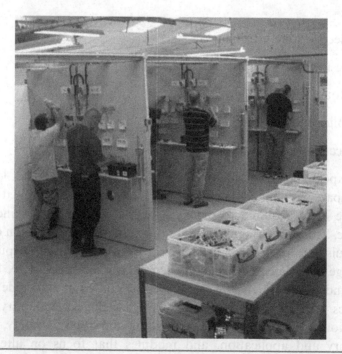

Figure 4.2 Many certified training programs include hands-on models.

You can also be considered qualified if you possess extensive knowledge, experience, and training, and have successfully demonstrated your ability to solve or resolve problems relating to the specific work or project to be performed. OSHA 1910.399 defines a qualified electrical worker as someone "who has received training in and has demonstrated skills and knowledge in the construction and operation of electric equipment and installations and the hazards involved." Since an OSHA defined qualified worker possesses training, certification, or extensive experience, OSHA 29 CFR 1926.651(f) requires that supporting systems design shall be by a qualified person.

SAFETY QUALIFIED

Both the NEC and OSHA describe qualified status as those who are trained in safe electrical installations. NFPA 70E Chapter 1 and OSHA 29 CFR 1910.331 through 1910.335 describe qualified workers as employees who are trained in and familiar with safety-related work practices. Since this is a broad statement, some clarification is in order. The question at hand is, what constitutes safety-related work practices? Here are some examples:

- The worker possesses the skills and techniques necessary to distinguish exposed live parts from the other parts of electric equipment.

- The employee has the skills and techniques necessary to determine the nominal voltage of exposed live parts.

- Electricians with knowledge of approach boundaries specified in NFPA 70E 130.2(C).

- Tradesmen with knowledge of hazard/risk category classifications specified in NFPA 70E 130.7(C)(9)(a).

- Employees with a comprehensive understanding of the personal protective equipment (PPE) matrix specified in NFPA 70E 130.7(C)(10) and protective clothing characteristics specified in NFPA 70E 130.7(C)(11).

- A person who is capable of working safely on energized circuits and who is familiar with the proper use of special precautionary techniques, PPE, insulating and shielding materials, and insulated tools.

- A tradesman who has documented skills and knowledge related to the construction and operation of the electrical equipment and installations and has received safety training on the hazards involved.

OSHA 1910.332(c) goes on to describe acceptable training as either classroom type or on-the-job type. The degree of training required is determined by the amount of risk posed to the employee (Figure 4.3).

Competent person

Qualified workers with safety training are not quite the same category as "competent" workers. OSHA 29 CFR 1926.32(f) and OSHA 1910.399 describe a competent person as someone who is capable of identifying existing and predictable hazards in the surroundings or working conditions which are hazardous or dangerous to employees, and who has the authorization to take prompt corrective measures to eliminate them (Figure 4.4).

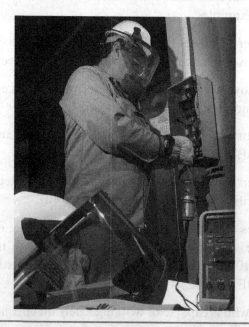

Figure 4.3 Employees who have safety hazard training are qualified to work on the systems that could possibly pose those hazards.

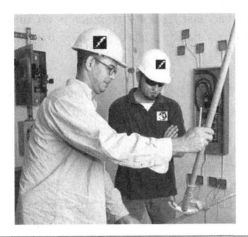

Figure 4.4 A competent person is trained to identify potential hazards caused by workmanship and site conditions.

This definition specifies that a competent person must have authority to take immediate action to eliminate hazards at the work site. For example, a competent person could be a job foreman whose role not only includes supervising electricians, but inspecting their work for code compliance, safe installation methods, and good workmanship. Job foremen typically make sure that wiring is the proper size and type, conduit is utilized where needed, GFI receptacles are included where required, and power systems are locked out and tagged out during installations to prevent exposure to energized systems. If the foreman is experienced enough to perform the same tasks as these electricians, and by the nature of his position has the authority to take corrective action as needed throughout the shift to ensure compliance through the control or elimination of hazards, then he is considered "competent." This is the reason a competent person is required under the inspection requirements outlined in OSHA 29 CFR 1926.650 and 29 CFR 1926.651.

Unqualified person

NFPA 70E article 100 requires that workers who might be exposed to an electrical hazard as a work task is performed must be trained to recognize that a hazard exists and how to avoid that hazard. Any person who has not received task specific training is an unqualified person. For example, you may be considered qualified to work near live parts, but not with live parts.

Based on NFPA 70E article 110, an unqualified person can work on non-energized electrical conductors, circuit parts, and de-energized equipment. To be considered de-energized means that electrical equipment is free from any electrical connection to a source of potential difference and from electrical charge; not having a potential different from that of the earth. The term de-energized describes an operating condition of electrical equipment and is not applicable to other power scenarios. De-energized does not guarantee a safe condition. This is one of the reasons that unqualified workers are required to be trained in and be familiar with electrical safety-related practices.

Let's look at a couple of situations where a person who is qualified to do certain tasks would be considered unqualified to perform other work. The three shock categories of approach boundaries include: limited, restricted, and prohibited. The limited, restricted, and prohibited approach boundaries are based on the voltage as illustrated in NFPA 70E Table 130.7(C)(9).

For an electrician to work within a limited approach boundary with exposed live parts he must be trained in all of the following:

- The skills and techniques necessary to distinguish exposed energized parts from other parts of electrical equipment

- The skills and techniques necessary to determine the nominal voltage of exposed live parts

- The decision-making process necessary to determine the degree and extent of the hazard and the PPE and job planning necessary to perform the task safely

- The appropriate PPE required

- The approach distances specified in Table 130.2(C) and the corresponding voltages to which the qualified person will be exposed

On the other hand, to be considered qualified to work within a restricted work boundary, an electrician must possess all of the skills above, have completed all required safety training, and have a written approved plan for the work to be performed, including shock-prevention procedures. He must plan the work to keep all parts of his body out of the area considered to be prohibited space (Figure 4.5).

A worker can be qualified to work near live parts but not within other types of established boundaries. For example, working near live parts involves any activity inside a limited approach boundary. The limited

Dimensions listed are the distance from energized electrical conductors or circuit part to the worker				
Nominal System Voltage Range, Phase to Phase	Limited Approach Boundary Exposed Movable Conductor3	Limited Approach Boundary Exposed Fixed Circuit Part	Restricted Approach Boundary, Includes Inadvertent Movement Factors	Prohibited Approach Boundary
Less than 50	Not specified	Not specified	Not specified	Not specified
50 to 300	10 ft 0 in.	3 ft 6 in.	Avoid contact	Avoid contact
301 to 750	10 ft 0 in.	3 ft 6 in.	1 ft 0 in.	0 ft 1 in.
751 to 15 kV	10 ft 0 in.	5 ft 0 in.	2 ft 2 in.	0 ft 7 in.
15.1 kV to 36 kV	10 ft 0 in.	6 ft 0 in.	2 ft 7 in.	0 ft 10 in.
36.1 kV to 46 kV	10 ft 0 in.	8 ft 0 in.	2 ft 9 in.	1 ft 5 in.
46.1 kV to 72.5 kV	10 ft 0 in.	8 ft 0 in.	3 ft 3 in.	2 ft 2 in.
72.6 kV to 121 kV	10 ft 8 in.	8 ft 0 in.	3 ft 4 in.	2 ft 9 in.
138 kV to 145 kV	11 ft 0 in.	10 ft 0 in.	3 ft 10 in.	3 ft 4 in.
161 kV to 169 kV	11 ft 8 in.	11 ft 8 in.	4 ft 3 in.	3 ft 9 in.
230 kV to 242 kV	13 ft 0 in.	13 ft 0 in.	5 ft 8 in.	5 ft 2 in.
345 kV to 362 kV	15 ft 4 in.	15 ft 4 in.	9 ft 2 in.	8 ft 8 in.
500 kV to 550 kV	19 ft 0 in.	19 ft 0 in.	11 ft 10 in.	11 ft 4 in.
765 kV to 800 kV	23 ft 9 in.	23 ft 9 in.	15 ft 11 in.	15 ft 5 in.

Figure 4.5   Approach boundaries are based on voltage and distance to energized parts.

approach boundary is the outermost boundary of any activity of a person working near live parts and cannot be crossed by an unqualified person unless that person is escorted by a qualified person. People may be outside the limited approach boundary but still be within the flash protection boundary, making them susceptible to second-degree burns. For this reason, workers must consider all of the hazards and how they are related to be properly protected and to determine who is considered unqualified.

As a qualified person, you need to know the difference between "live parts," which are energized conductive components, and "exposed" parts, which are capable of being inadvertently touched if approached closer than a safe distance by a person. Exposed parts are not suitably guarded, isolated, or insulated.

ENERGIZED WORK ANALYSIS AND PERMITS

Energized work, or hot work, can only be performed by qualified personnel. NFPA 70E is very specific regarding justifiable conditions that can prompt hot work. Whenever feasible, energized parts greater than 50 V to which an employee might be exposed need to be put into an electrically safe work condition before an employee works on or near them (Figure 4.6).

ELECTRICALLY SAFE WORK CONDITION

In order to prevent exposure to electrical hazards all sources of energy must be removed and isolated from the system. With no source of electrical energy present, an electrical hazard is not present and consequently requirements for energized electrical work do not apply.

IMPORTANT NOTE: the acts of opening a disconnecting means, measuring for the absence of voltage, visually verifying a physical break in the power conductors, and installing safety grounds all contain a risk of injury. Since these actions are necessary to achieve an electrically safe work condition, they must be performed by a qualified person wearing personal protective equipment based on the degree of potential hazard.

Figure 4.6 Creating electrically safe work conditions poses some risks.

Diagnostic work such as troubleshooting or testing where the equipment or system must be energized in order to perform the testing is justifiable by its nature and does not require energize work documentation. All safe work practices, including appropriate PPE and tools as determined by a hazard assessment, must be used.

Work that is not for diagnostic purposes and does not allow for the equipment or system to be put into an electrically safe work condition must be justified in writing by using an energized electrical work analysis. In order to rationalize this type of work, you must demonstrate that de-energizing the system actually introduces additional or increased hazards, or is infeasible due to equipment design or operational limitations. While the process of removing and isolating energy from electrical systems ensures safe working conditions, it is often a time-consuming and inconvenient process. The terms infeasible and inconvenient are significantly different, and the two terms are not used interchangeably. Mere inconvenience cannot serve to justify work on or near exposed live parts. Work by a qualified person on or near exposed live parts is only justifiable under the following conditions:

1. When de-energizing the conductors or equipment would result in an increased or additional hazard. For instance, if placing the power system of a nursing home or hospital in an electrically safe work condition would disconnect electrical power to life support equipment. Another scenario would be if the absence of electrical power could result in an environmental spill, deactivation of emergency alarm systems in an occupied building, or the shutdown of hazardous location ventilation equipment that is in use.

2. If de-energizing the conductors or equipment is not feasible because of the nature of equipment design or operational limitations. A typical situation would be when diagnostics and testing, such as start-up or troubleshooting, can only be performed with the circuit energized. Additionally, work on circuits that form an integral part of a continuous process that would otherwise need to be completely shut down in order to permit work on one circuit or piece of equipment, such as in a chemical processing plant.

It is important to note that lack of illumination is not justification for live work. If de-energizing a system means you would be working in the dark, then temporary lighting must be installed. For voltages that are less than 50 V, the decision to de-energize a system should include consideration of the energy source and any overcurrent protection between the energy source and the worker. Even electrical energy less than 50 V can be hazardous. For example, control circuits that operate at less than 50 V could impact processes that result in a release of another kind of energy. So even if the capacity of the energy source is limited, the integrity of the circuit must be considered as well.

Electrical work involving multi-wire branch circuits must be treated as energized work whenever it is necessary to break the continuity of the grounded conductor.

When it is necessary to perform work on energized equipment, OSHA 1910.333(a)(2) requires that safety-related work practices must be used. To comply with safe practices, the person performing the work must be qualified and trained in the selection of PPE. For hot work, you should use the appropriate PPE in dry run to make sure the PPE selected does not limit your dexterity or vision. NFPA 70E article 110 states that work on energized electrical conductors and circuits may only be performed by qualified workers. If the energized electrical conductors or circuit parts cannot be placed in an electrically safe work condition, safety-related work practices must be used that protect employees from arc flash and from contact with energized electrical conductors or circuit parts operating at 50 V or more directly with any part of their body or indirectly through some other conductive object.

Safe work practices are demonstrated by documenting the rationale, purpose, and process for energized work by using an energized work analysis. NFPA suggests that this assessment should identify the purpose of the task and the qualifications of and number of employees needed to perform the task. The hazards and scope of the task should be described and sketches or electrical diagrams can be used to explain the task and the safe work practices to be used. It is essential to include approach distances, PPE that will be used, and insulating materials and tools that will be utilized.

NFPA 70E article 110 also requires you to perform a shock hazard analysis to determine the voltage workers will be exposed to and associated boundary requirements.

NFPA 70E article 130 provides Table 130.2C which lists the acceptable approach boundaries to energized electrical conductors or circuits parts for shock protection. The limited approach boundary described in the table is the closest approach distance for an unqualified worker (unless additional protective measures are used). The restrictive approach boundary is the closest approach distance for a qualified person, and the prohibited approach boundary is the distance that should not be encroached unless the work task is guided by the measures listed in NFAP 70E Section 130.1.

Energized electrical work assessment

A safety hazard analysis provides detailed information regarding the hazards you expect to encounter and protective measures that you will use prior to beginning any hot work.

A shock hazard assessment is done to determine the voltage personnel will be exposed to and a flash hazard analysis establishes the appropriate rating of the clothing and PPE to be used as well as the location of any arc-flash boundary (Figure 4.7).

DANGER: If the flash hazard analysis indicates that the intensity of a potential arc flash could expose a worker to 40 calories per square centimeter (cal/cm2), hot work **must not** be performed. This is because there is no protective equipment that exists that can protect the worker from the intense pressure produced by an arcing fault with an intensity greater than 40 cal/cm2.

Figure 4.7 PPE cannot protect against all potential hazards.

Energized work permits

Energized work permits are used to document your intention to perform hot work and your client's understanding of the scope of work that will be done. Unlike the usual permits obtained from local municipalities that enable you to work on property within a town or city, this is a permit that you will generate.

The energized electrical work permit proves to your client and OSHA that you have thoroughly planned out the need and process for working on energized electrical circuits. In the event that there is an accident, you will need to provide the information in this document to OSHA. As you are filling out this form, signing it, and writing your justifications, you gain a clear understanding of what an OSHA compliance officer would look for if any problems or incidents occur.

A sample form is provided in the appendix section of NFPA 70E. NFPA 70E requires that, "if live parts are not placed into an electrically safe work condition... work to be performed shall be considered energized electrical work and shall be performed by written permit only." An exception provides for work performed on or near live parts by a qualified person. If this work is related to tasks such as testing, troubleshooting, voltage measuring, etc., it can be performed without an energized electrical work permit provided appropriate safe work practices and PPE is provided and used. The reason this exception makes sense, is that "work" is defined as installing or moving energized conductors, whereas "testing and troubleshooting" generally involves touching an instrument or probe to the energized conductor. If you perform service work in a commercial environment, troubleshooting is something you do often. Just be advised that while an energized work permit is not required, a hazard analysis is. The reason for this is that the hazard still exists, even if the risk of contact is reduced.

NFPA 70E spells out what has to be included in an energized work permit. It should include, but is not limited to, the following items:

- A description of the circuit and equipment to be worked on and the location

- The name and qualifications of the person or people who will be performing the work

- The start date and time and the estimated finish date and time for the job

- Justification/rationale for why the work must be performed in an energized condition

- A description of the safe work practices that will be used

- Results of the shock hazard analysis

- Determination of the shock protection boundaries

- Results of the flash hazard analysis

- The flash protection boundary

- The necessary PPE to safely perform the assigned task

- Methods that will be used to restrict the access of unqualified persons from the work area

- A copy of a job briefing that included an explanation of any job-specific hazards

- Signature of approval from the property owner, safety officer, manager, or other authorized individual

When you are describing the work to be done, consider the working conditions that are present as well. Some examples of these associated conditions and potential hazards are:

- Existing electrical conditions that could pose a hazard, such as massive grounds that may be adjacent to the work, or live input/output terminals. Other energized circuits close by that may have different voltage, be a different phase, or require different lockout locations for de-energizing.

- Mechanical conditions such as rotating equipment, shear hazards of the equipment or adjacent equipment, other equipment that can and needs to be de-energized or locked out.

- Environmental conditions including flammable vapors, combustible materials, or any other type of physical or biological hazards.

- Working space constraints that make access to the equipment limited or difficult, including energized circuits or parts that will be present behind the qualified work, or irregular or uneven working surfaces. Include an assessment of obstructions that could make emergency escape difficult.

The benefits of completing an energized electrical work permit really do outweigh the inconvenience associated with producing it. It is a tool for planning out the work as well as documentation of the justification for the hot work. The permit can be used in a job briefing to communicate to your coworkers the rationale behind working energized. Since part of the permit involves performing a hazard assessment, the permit also acts as an aid to selecting the proper PPE necessary for your protection from shock and arc flash hazards. Defining work boundaries results in safety precautions that will keep unqualified workers out of harms way. One of the most beneficial aspects of using the permit is that it provides approval to perform the work energized. Since the work has to be authorized, a representative for the property is involved and completely informed of the risks and reasons for the work and can assist with additional information or preparation critical to the work. When work must be done energized, using an energized electrical work permit will help you prepare to face the work hazards ahead with a level of professionalism, productivity, and safety.

LOCKOUT/TAGOUT

The term "lockout/tagout" describes procedures used to safeguard employees from the unexpected energization or startup of machinery and equipment, or the release of hazardous energy during service, maintenance, or installation of additional equipment.

Approximately 3 million workers a year risk injury if lockout/tagout is not properly utilized. Lockout/tagout is responsible for preventing an estimated 120 fatalities and 50,000 injuries annually. Workers injured on the job from exposure to hazardous energy lose an average of 24 workdays for recuperation, so it's no surprise that OSHA, NFPA, and the NEC all require the implementation of safe precautions to de-energize equipment before working on it. Lockout/tagout, or lock and tag, is a recognized safety practice that is used to ensure that dangerous machines are properly shut off and cannot be started up again prior to the completion of maintenance or servicing work. The procedure requires that hazardous power sources are "isolated and rendered inoperative" before any kind of repair work is performed. The lockout/tagout process utilizes a lock that isolates the designated device or the power source and places it in an "off" position that prohibits hazardous power sources from being turned on. Additionally, a tag is attached to the locking means that identifies the name of the worker who de-energized and locked the power source and indicates that the device must not be turned on (Figure 4.8).

When two or more subcontractors are working on different parts of a larger overall system, the locked-out device is first secured with a folding scissors clamp that has numerous padlock holes capable of holding it closed. Then each subcontractor applies his own padlock to the clamp. In this way, the locked-out device cannot be activated until all of the affected workers have signed off on their portion of the project and removed their padlock from the clamp. Each lock should have its own unique key so that no two keys or locks are the same.

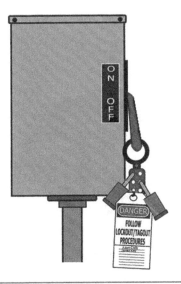

Figure 4.8 A multiple lock device is signed by each person who affixes a lock.

Furthermore, a person's lock and tag must not be removed by anyone other than the individual who installed the lock and tag. It's not uncommon for a facility to have several energy sources that need to be de-energized, including the device itself, upstream material feeders, and downstream feeders. When more than one crew is involved, overall job coordination and safety control is managed by the "person-in-charge." This term is used to describe one qualified person who is designated as an authorized employee with overall responsibility for the lockout procedure. Utilizing a multiple lock system that is managed by a single supervisor ensures the safety of everyone working on related parts of the same system (Figure 4.9).

Safety equipment manufacturers make a wide range of isolation devices that are specifically designed to fit a variety of switches, valves, and effectors. For example, most modern circuit breakers are made to allow a small padlock to be attached to lock the breakers in the OFF position. For other devices such as ball or gate valves, there are plastic pieces that fit against the pipe and prevent movement, or clam shell-style locks that surround the valve and prevent its use. A common feature of lockout devices is that they are brightly colored, often red, to increase visibility and enable workers to easily identify that a device is isolated. Locks are also designed to prevent them being removed by force.

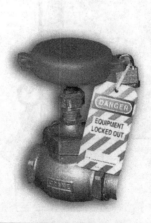

Figure 4.9 Some lockout devices are made to secure motor-operated valves.

One of the hazards associated with "locking out" such items as electrical disconnects is unless you open the cover to assure that all blades have broken contact, the circuit is still energized.

The National Electrical Code has general requirements that require that a safety service disconnect must be installed within sight of the serviceable equipment. To qualify as "within sight," the disconnect must be obvious, easy to see, and not more than 50 feet from the equipment that will be worked on. OSHA compliance standards addressing lockout/tagout requirements include OSHA 29 CFR 1910.147 and 926 Subpart K, Electrical 1926.417, which establish an employer's responsibility to protect employees from hazardous energy sources on machines and equipment during service and maintenance.

The standard outlines the steps required to do this, which include the following:

- Employers must develop, document, implement, and enforce an energy control program.

- Lockout devices must be used for equipment that can be locked out. Tagout devices may be used instead of lockout devices only if the tagout means provides protection for employees that is equivalent to that provided through a lockout system.

- Employers and business owners have to ensure that new or overhauled equipment is capable of being locked out.

- Use only lockout/tagout devices that are authorized or made specifically for the particular equipment, machinery, or application and that are durable, standardized, and substantial.

- Ensure that lockout/tagout devices have a means to identify individual users.

- Establish a safety policy that only allows the employee who applied a lockout/tagout device to remove it.

- Inspect energy control procedures at least annually and provide effective training for all of the employees covered by the standard.

- Comply with associated energy control provisions in OSHA standards when machines or equipment need to be tested or repositioned, when outside contractors work at the site, in group lockout situations, and during shift or personnel changes.

Stored energy

Stored energy is the residual or built-up energy held within a component. The easiest way to visualize stored energy is to associate it with cutting the water off in your house. When you shut the main water supply off in your home, there is no new water source coming into the lines, but if you open one of the faucets, built-up water will still be released. This continues until the hydraulic pressure pushes out all of the stored water in the plumbing lines. Electrical energy works in much the same way.

Stored energy can occur in capacitors or batteries, or in spring-loaded devices, suspended weights, or compressed gases. This is easy to remember if you have ever tested a household battery by putting it on your tongue. If you get a tingling zap, the battery is not completely dead. Just because the flashlight that you took the battery out of was not lighting up does not mean all of the batteries in it were completely empty. This risk is amplified with equipment and machinery, capacitors, and condensers. Stored electrical energy must be dissipated by discharging or grounding after the main energy source has been isolated. Carefully release all stored energy as part of the de-energizing process and be mindful that many types of machinery contain more than one energy source.

Test to make sure that all stored energy has been released. Push the start button on equipment to verify that all electrical energy is eliminated and has been properly deactivated or isolated. Try the on-off switch, not the isolation switch, or attempt to operate other controls to be sure the machine won't start. This verifies that all stored energy has been released.

Stored energy hazards occur when energy that is confined is released unexpectedly. This hazard is present in pressurized systems and their components, including springs, hydraulic, pneumatic, and electrical systems. Before you lockout electrical systems, you must make sure that all equipment is completely free of electricity.

Types of lockout/tagout

There are two types of lockout/tagout procedures. The first is a simple system that requires the person-in-charge to notify all affected employees/workers before the application and after the removal of lockout/tagout devices. An authorized employee has to shutdown the equipment to be worked on using procedures that have been established for the equipment or power sources. Additionally, the person-in-charge is responsible for confirming that all hazardous energy sources are controlled and that all authorized employees working on the system attach individual locks during the lockout process. Finally, the person-in-charge must verify that all locks have been removed and that the equipment has been properly re-energized.

COMPLEX LOCKOUT/TAGOUT

One of the most significant differences between simple lockout and complex lockout/tagout is that complex or group lockout/tagout requires written plans or procedures. The written plan needs to define the requirements for the person-in-charge and identify affected and authorized workers. The person-in-charge has the primary responsibility for directly implementing a complex lockout/tagout procedure and therefore accepts responsibility as the primary authorized employee/worker. The person-in-charge should implement the following processes:

Step 1   Follow the written complex lockout/tagout plan which should include:

■ A specific statement of intent of use;

■ Specific procedural steps for isolating, blocking, and securing machines or equipment for hazardous energy or material;

■ Specific steps for testing to verify the absence of hazardous energy;

■ Procedures for affixing and removing lockout/tagout devices;

■ Parties who are responsible for locks and tags and their proper working condition;

- Specific requirements for testing machines and equipment to verify the effectiveness of all lockout/tagout control measures. This should include turning equipment off.

Step 2 The responsible employee for each crew, trade, or group must ensure that all the people working under their lock are trained in and familiar with the lockout/tagout process. This includes being informed of the type, magnitude, and sources of hazardous energy, control methods, and a list of personnel to be notified when the responsible employee removes their lock.

Step 3 The person-in-charge must ensure that all affected employees/workers are notified before the application and after the removal of lockout/tagout.

Step 4 The equipment operator or an authorized worker is responsible for shutting down the affected equipment using the procedures established for the machine or equipment.

Step 5 After de-energization, the person-in-charge must verify that all sources of hazardous energy have been controlled to minimize exposure to all workers.

Step 6 Each authorized employee working on the task must attach his/her own individual lock. NOTE: if an energy-isolating device is capable of being locked, a lock must be used.

Step 7 A tag for the person-in-charge is required in addition to locks, and must clearly indicate the company and employee applying the lock, if this information is not contained on the lock.

Step 8 If an energy isolating device is not capable of being locked, tagout devices must be affixed to clearly indicate that the operation of the energy isolating device is prohibited and additional means must be used, including the implementation of additional safety measures such as the removal of an isolating circuit element, blocking controlling switches, opening any extra disconnecting devices, etc.

Step 9 Upon completion of work, the person-in-charge must confirm the proper removal of all locks and tags.

Step 10 Following the removal of all locks and tags, the person-in-charge must confirm that all equipment is returned to the "on" position and oversee the re-energization of all equipment.

LOCKOUT/TAGOUT SAVES LIVES

All of these steps—documentation, checking, and verifying—may seem like far more trouble than they are worth. The reality is that electricity can kill or maim you and the effects of electrocution are devastating. Maybe you'll be sufficiently motivated to go through the inconvenience of locking out power by reading Mike's story.

Mike is a journeyman electrician who worked for the commercial electrical contractor where I was the safety and human resources director. On a Friday Mike went to the shopping center remodel job where he had been working all week. The night before, the power had been left off at the panel and the precautionary locks were removed. Mike's first task of the day was to go up on the scissor lift and trim out a few remaining light fixtures. The job supervisor, who was the person-in-charge, checked to make sure that the power was still off at the panel and went on to trim out some receptacles. Meanwhile, an electrician who was assigned to the job for the first time arrived and went into the back of the store to unpack fixtures, but the room was dim because no lights were on. He flipped on the light switch and when nothing happened he went to the power panel and turned on the main and all of the breakers that were labeled "lights." What happened next would change Mike's life forever.

Holding his wire stripper in his right hand and the light fixture wires in his left, Mike's body was suddenly shocked with 220 V of continuous electricity and he let out a blood-curdling scream. His muscles constricted, he was unable to let go of the hot wires, and his wire stripper tipped down on his left hand as his right hand convulsed. At the same time, the job foreman saw lights come on in the building and ran to the power panel to throw the main breaker. Once the power was cut, Mike's body collapsed on the deck of the scissor lift and he didn't move. The supervisor tried to lower the lift, but the electrical shock had shorted the controls. Two workers scaled the sides of the lift, while several others began to manually lower the lift. When they got to Mike he was still unconscious, and by the time the ambulance arrived he was awake but disoriented. Both of his hands were covered with blisters and he was taken directly to the cardiovascular unit of the hospital. His heart was monitored overnight to make sure that it had not been damaged and his hand injuries were treated. Unfortunately, his wire strippers had burned through two of his fingers down to the bone and the attending physician was convinced that they would have to be amputated (Figure 4.10).

For the next year Mike fought to save his fingers and regain the use of both of his hands. He went to physical therapy, had his left hand surgically attached to his waste to graft live tissue to his damaged fingers, and underwent tendon replacement surgery. He lost months of work,

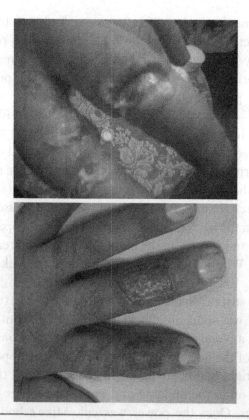

Figure 4.10 Mike's fingers were burned through to the bone as a result of 220 V of electricity shocking his body.

endured painful debriding of dead flesh over and over again, and still has scars on his hands. He continues to suffer from muscle pain in his hands and arms, which has been attributed to deep tissue death, but in the end, Mike was thrilled just to be alive and to have some use of his left hand. One painless action could have prevented all this trauma—affixing a lock to the energized power panel.

All lockout/tagout procedures, whether they are simple or complex, require pre-planning, caution, and attention to detail. Always confirm your lockout/tagout and retest for the absence of energy if conditions change, or, as in the case of Mike's story, when the job location has been left unattended, be sure to inform all workers that lockout procedures are in place.

Re-energizing protocols

After the work or maintenance is complete and equipment is ready for normal operations, the authorized employee needs to first clear the area around the machines or equipment of all personnel to ensure that no one is exposed during re-energizing. Additionally, the area needs to be cleared of any tools, miscellaneous materials, ladders, toolboxes, etc. After these items have been removed from the space around the machine or equipment, any guards need to be reinstalled and the equipment should be placed back in the "on" position. Next, the person-in-charge can safely remove lockout devices. If multiple locks have been attached during the lockout process, each person who attached a lock must be present to remove his own lock. This step is essential to guard against injury, because it requires the owner of the lock to notify their workers that circuits or equipment are about to be energized. Think of this as "no man (or woman) left behind" in the chain of re-energizing power. After all of these steps have been taken, the authorized employee can operate the energy-isolating devices to restore energy to the machine or equipment.

One of your best safety practices is to be proactive against existing and potential electrical hazards. This happens through knowledge, awareness, experience, and practicing safety protocols. When working with electricity, an ounce of prevention or taking the time to exercise a few additional work steps is worth its weight in saved costs, personal safety, and job completion (Figure 4.00).

Lockout/Tagout Safety Quiz

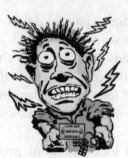

1. Place numbers from 1 to 7 in the correct order of a lockout/tagout process

___ Isolate equipment
___ Verify isolation
___ Control stored energy
___ Shut down equipment
___ Prepare for shutdown
___ Apply lockout/tagout devices
___ Removal of locks

TRUE of FALSE: check whether each of the following questions is True or is False:

2. The Lockout/Tagout process is used to ensure that equipment you've isolated and de-energized remains shut down. True___ or False___

3. During a tagout, a tag is placed on all primary and secondary energy sources. True___ or False___

4. Equipment is rendered in a safe condition once the power has been shut down. True___ or False___

5. A pre-job briefing should be held with all co-workers before a lockout operation. True___ or False___

6. You can remove locks if your co-worker gives you the keys. True___ or False___

7. Kinetic energy is the energy in an object when it is in motion. True___ or False___

8. In preparing for a shutdown, gravity is not a consideration. True___ or False___

MULTIPLE CHOICE: Circle all of the answers that are correct for each of the following questions:

9. Which of the following must you know before starting to work on a piece of equipment.
a) magnitude of energy to be controlled, b) hazards of energy to be controlled, c) types of energy to be controlled, d) method and means to control the energy,

10. Which of the following people must be notified prior to shutting down equipment for repair? a) plant manager, b) supervisor, c) safety person, d) affected employees.

11. Which of the following would be involved in equipment isolation? a) closing valves, b) locking out feeders, c) turning off power, d) releasing hydraulic pressure, e) releasing steam pressure, f) blocking movement of parts, g) releasing spring tension.

12. Locks are located at which of the following: a) electric panel, b) switch, c) water valve, d) isolating device.

13. Which of the following would be part of control of stored energy? a) closing valves, b) locking out feeders, c) turning off power, d) releasing hydraulic pressure, e) releasing steam pressure, f) blocking movement of parts, g) releasing spring tension.

14. Verifying isolation involves which of the following actions: a) putting locks on the equipment, b) putting a tag on the equipment, c) attempting to turn the machine on.

Answers

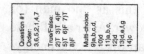

Question #1 Order:	True/False:	Multi-choice:
3,6,5,2,1,4,7	2)T 3)T 4)F	9)a,b,c,d
	5)T 6)F 7)T	10)d
	8)F	11)a,b,c,
		12)d
		13)d,e,f,g
		14)c

Figure 4.00 A Lock Out Tag Out quiz such as this can be incorporated into your safety trainings as a means of documenting working awareness.

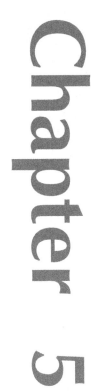

Electrical System Grounding and Bonding

Chapter Outline

Doi: 10.1016/B978-1-85617-654-5.00005-4

When you are working on electrical installations, the earth is one of your best safety devices. You may not think of the earth as a device, but when you ground electrical circuits to the earth, it can protect you by diverting dangerous current away from you and into the ground. For this simple reason, in the language of electricians the term "ground" literally means earth.

Terms to know

Article 100 and Article 250 of the National Electrical Code provides a number of definitions regarding grounding and bonding. Let's take a minute to review them.

- *Bonded (bonding):* Connected in a manner so as to establish electrical continuity and conductivity.

- *Bonding jumper, main:* The connection between the grounded circuit conductor and the equipment grounding conductor (EGC) at an electrical service.

- *Equipment grounding conductor:* A conductive path that is installed to connect the normally non-current-carrying metal parts of equipment together and also to the system grounded conductor, the grounding electrode conductor, or both.

- *Ground:* The earth.

- *Grounded (grounding):* Connected to the ground or to conductive material that extends the ground connection.

- *Grounded conductor:* A system or circuit conductor that is intentionally grounded.

- *Grounding conductor:* A conductor that is used to connect equipment or the grounded circuit of a wiring system to a grounding electrode.

- *Grounding electrode conductor:* A conductor that is used to connect the system grounded conductor of the equipment to the grounding electrode or to a point on the grounding electrode system.

■ *Ground fault:* The unintentional, electrical conductor connection between an ungrounded circuit conductor and normally non-current carrying conductors, metallic enclosures, metallic raceways, metallic equipment, or the earth.

■ *Ground-fault current path:* An electrically conductive path from the point of a ground-fault on a wiring system through normally non-current carrying conductors, equipment, or the earth to the electrical supply source.

What is grounding?

A "ground" is a conductive connection between an electrical circuit or a piece of equipment and the earth or another type of conductive material that is used in place of the earth. Both OSHA and the NEC have very specific requirements for utilizing grounding to reduce the risk of injury. The rationale for these requirements is simple—all electrical installations have to provide a means of transferring electrical current in the event of a circuit fault to reduce potential shock hazards (Figure 5.1).

Grounding protects against shock hazards posed by fault currents. An electrical fault occurs when current flows through an abnormal or unintended path. For example, if the insulation in a conductor is damaged, the means of containing and directing the electrical current running through it will be compromised and ineffective. A fault current is several times greater than the current that normally flows through a circuit, because it is essentially electricity running wild instead of flowing in a controlled manner. Electricity always follows the path of least resistance, and that path could be you if a fault occurs within electrical equipment or components that have not been grounded.

There are three basic reasons for grounding:

■ To limit voltage surges caused by lightning, utility system operations, or accidental contact with high-voltage lines

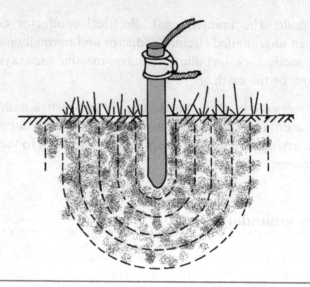

Figure 5.1 Grounding is a means of connecting electrical circuits to the earth.

- To provide a connect to the earth that can stabilize voltage under normal operating conditions
- To facilitate the operation of overcurrent devices such as circuit breakers, fuses, and relays under ground-fault conditions

All 120- and 240-volt circuits need to have a system of grounding. Grounding assures that all metal parts of a circuit that you might come in contact with are connected directly to the earth, maintaining them at zero voltage. Grounding directs electrical energy into the earth by providing a conductor that is less resistant than you are. Grounding is achieved by attaching one end of a conductor wire to the frame of a piece of equipment, panel, or appliance and the other end to a ground conductor. This conductor provides the connection to the earth needed to properly transfer electrical current in case of a fault.

The National Electrical Code addresses grounding of systems that are required to be connected to the earth in NEC 250.4(A). In order to limit the voltage to ground, any non-current carrying materials that are conductive and enclose electrical equipment or conductors have to be connected to the earth. There is a fine print note (FPN) in the 2008 edition of NEC Section 250.4 that encourages you to minimize the length of the grounding electrode conductor by calling your attention to NEC Sections 800.100(A)(5), 810.21(E), and 820.100(A)(5) that require grounding conductors to be run as short and as straight as possible. This results in the most effective path to the earth for line surges caused by lightning events.

Ground faults versus short circuits

A short circuit is an unintentional connection between two conductors that could be either phase-to-phase or phase-to-neutral. A ground fault is an unintentional connection between an ungrounded, or "phase," conductor and a conductive material such as a metal enclosure or raceway, or metal equipment frame. Short circuits are not too common because two insulation failures would have to occur for the unintentional connection to take place. In this kind of situation, an overcurrent device such as a circuit breaker should protect the circuit by opening quickly. Ground faults, on the other hand, are more common because a ground fault only requires a single insulation failure. A ground fault can be much more destructive than a short circuit. If you do not install a code-compliant ground-fault current return path, the result could be a high-impedance arcing fault that lasts a long time without causing a circuit breaker to trip or a fuse to blow (Figure 5.2).

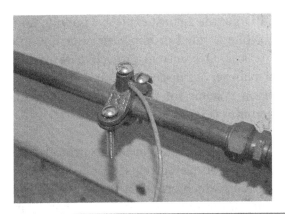

Figure 5.2 Copper water pipe can serve as an effective ground-fault current path.

The NEC makes a distinction between just a ground-fault current path and an effective ground-fault current path. A ground-fault current path is any conductive material that fault current can flow through. These conductive means are not limited to conductors or equipment. They can include water lines or gas pipes, air ducts, communications wiring, fences, rain gutters, and so on. An effective ground-fault current path is an intentionally designed and constructed low-impedance route that is meant to carry ground-fault current. In other words, a ground-fault current path can be accidental, but an effective ground-fault current path is always an intentional and critical element of an electrical grounding and bonding system. NEC Section 250.4(A)(5) requires that an effective ground-fault current path must be permanent, low-impedance, and able to carry the maximum ground-fault current that is likely to be imposed on it from any point on the wiring system. It does not consider the earth as an "effective" ground-fault current path, only because the earth's resistance is high enough that hardly any fault current returns to the electrical supply source through the earth. For this reason, the code requires that EGCs have to be run with circuit conductors to be deemed effectively grounded.

Overcurrent protection devices

Overcurrent protection is critical to personal safety and protection from a number of hazardous conditions that can result from materials igniting due to improper overload protection or short-circuit protection. Additionally, the OCPD guards against explosive ignition and flash hazards from inadequate voltage-rated or improper interrupting-rated overcurrent protective devices. Overcurrent protective devices, or OCPDs, are typically used in main service disconnects, and in the feeders and branch circuits of electrical systems for residential, commercial, institutional, and industrial premises (Figure 5.3).

Overcurrent protection devices are meant to protect against the potentially dangerous effects of overcurrents, such as an overload current or a short-circuit current, which creates a fault current. Equipment damage, personal injury, and even death can result from the improper application of a device's voltage rating, current rating, or interrupting rating.

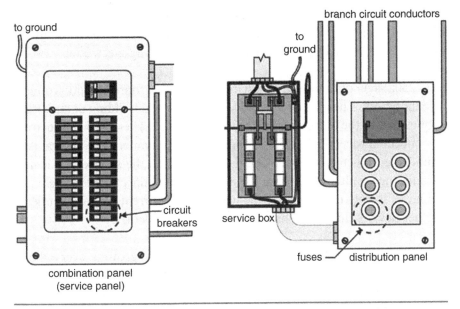

Figure 5.3 Overcurrent protection devices include circuit breakers and fuses.

Something as simple as a circuit breaker can protect against this damage, but if a fuse or circuit breaker doesn't have an adequate voltage rating, it can rupture or explode while attempting to stop fault currents beyond their interrupting ratings. Grounding helps to protect against inadequate overcurrent protection or OCPD failure. The two processes are designed to work together to protect equipment, property, and people.

Grounded versus grounding

Throughout code regulations there are terms that appear very similar such as "grounding" and "grounded," but the distinction between them is very important to your safety and to hazard-free installations. When the term grounded is used by itself it describes a connection to the earth or a conductive material that extends the connection to the earth. So it makes sense that a grounded conductor is a circuit conductor that is intentionally connected to the earth. Neutrals are one type of grounded conductor, and grounded conductors are color coded with either a white or gray outer finish. Yet, a grounding conductor is specifically used to connect equipment or the grounded circuit of a wiring system to the earth. These conductors can and should be bare, covered, or insulated and are connected to the earth by a grounding electrode.

NEC 250.24(A) outlines the installation order for grounded and grounding conductors. The grounded conductor system of a building or structure is connected to the feeder conductors at the service. These two conductors are connected together by using a main bonding jumper. The neutral is a grounded conductor by virtue of the connection at the service, but is not a grounding conductor because it is not used to connect anything else to ground. It is only used to carry the normal load current of lights, outlets, or other devices that are connected from phase to neutral.

The grounded conductor remains isolated from ground everywhere except for the bond at the service. If more than one connection to ground is made, load neutral currents will divide between the grounded conductor and the EGCs. This can result in continuous current flow on conduit systems or metal structures and piping, which can cause electrolytic corrosion and interference with sensitive electronic equipment due to radiated magnetic fields.

NEC 250.26 lists the specifications for AC system grounding conductors. These are listed in the table below (Figure 5.4):

GROUNDING ELECTRODES

A grounding electrode is the actual device that establishes the electrical connection to the earth, such as a rod driven into the earth. Typically, two or more grounding electrodes will be interconnected and connected

| NEC 250.26 Requires AC Premise Wiring System Grounded Conductors ||
Type of System	Conductor To Be Used
Single Phase 2-Wire	One Conductor
Single Phase 3-Wire	The Neutral Conductor
Multiphase with One Wire Common To All Phases	The Common Conductor
Multiphase with One Grounded Phase	One Phase Conductor
Multiphase with One Phase Used as a Single Phase 3-Wire	The Neutral Conductor

Figure 5.4 AC conductors that are grounded must be specified in the manner listed.

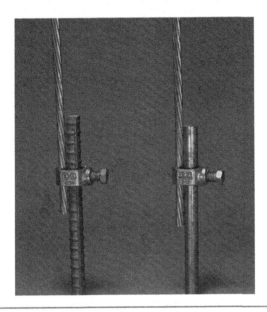

Figure 5.5 Grounded electrodes.

to the service neutral by the grounding electrode conductor. The grounding electrode is used to maintain conductors connected to it at ground potential and also to dissipate current conducted to it into the earth (Figure 5.5).

A grounding electrode is any of a number of devices that establishes an electrical connection to the earth. There are several vehicles for forming this connection as follows:

- A metal underground pipe
- The metal frame of a building
- A concrete-encased electrode
- A ground ring that encircles the building
- Rod and pipe electrodes
- Plate electrodes

Each of these electrode methods has specific requirements. For example, interior metal water pipes must be located within 5 feet of the point of entrance to a building in order to be used as grounding electrodes. The metal frame of a building must have 10 feet or more of structural direct contact to the earth or be encased in concrete that is in direct contact with the earth in order to meet the standard for a grounding electrode.

A ground rod must be buried at least 8 feet in the ground.

NEC requirements for a concrete-encased electrode include vertical electrodes and instructions on what to do when multiple isolated concrete-encased electrodes are present. Structural steel rebar in vertical foundations is considered suitable as a grounding electrode, as long as it meets all of the requirements for horizontal structural steel rebar electrodes. Additionally, a building with multiple isolated concrete-encased electrodes, such as for spot footings, is only required to use one of these "present" electrodes. All of the concrete-encased electrodes to be bonded together would not provide any greater safeguard than using just one electrode.

Pipes or conduit used as electrodes must have a diameter of at least ¾ inch trade size, iron or steel rods need to be at least ⅝ inch trade size, stainless steel rods cannot be less than ⅝ inch in diameter, and nonferrous rods need to be at least ½ inch in diameter. If a grounding ring is used as an electrode, it must encircle the building and be in direct contact with the earth. Additionally, this type of electrode must consist of at least 20 feet of bare copper conductor that is at least #2 AWG.

If more than one of the permissible types of electrode systems are used, then each electrode in the grounding electrode system has to be within 6 feet of the other, unless the grounding electrodes are bonded together, in which case they are considered to be a single grounding electrode system.

There are two types of electrodes that are specifically not allowed to be used as grounding electrodes. These are metal underground gas pipe systems and aluminum electrodes.

GROUNDING ELECTRODE CONDUCTORS

Once you understand the purpose and applications of a ground electrode, you will be able to see the difference between the ground electrode and grounding electrode conductors. A grounding electrode conductor is used to connect a system grounded conductor from equipment to the grounding electrode or to a point on the grounding electrode system. The grounding electrode conductor connects the neutral of the power source to the earth and terminates in one or more grounding electrodes. This conductor's job is to provide a low-impedance connection from earth to the neutral as a return path for current should a circuit supplied from the service inadvertently contact earth or a structure connected to earth. The conductor size is specified based on the size of the service entrance conductors, and it is required to be installed continuously without splices.

Not just any conductor will work as a grounded electrode conductor. Table 250.66 in the NEC lists the minimum sizes for the grounded electrode conductors of grounded or ungrounded AC systems, as well as to derived conductors of separately derived AC systems. The table deals strictly with the size of the largest ungrounded service-entrance conductor or the equal area for parallel conductors, and specifies the minimum size of the grounding electrode conductor (Figure 5.6).

Minimum Required Size of Grounding Electrode Conductors		Size of the Largest Ungrounded Service-Entrance Conductor/ Equivalent Parallel Conductor Area	
Copper (AWG)	Aluminum or Copper-Clad Aluminum (AWG)	Copper (AWG)	Aluminum or Copper-Clad Aluminum (AWG)
8	6	2 or smaller	1/0 or smaller
6	4	1 or 1/0	2/0 or 3/0
4	2	2/0 or 3/0	4/0 or 250
2	1/0	Over 3/0 but less than 350	Over 250 to 500
1/0	3/0	Over 350 but less than 600	Over 500 to 900
2/0	4/0	Over 600 but less than 1100	Over 900 to 1750
3/0	250	Over 1100	Over 1750

Figure 5.6   The minimum size of these conductors is not based on the application of the grounding electrode.

If multiple sets of service-entrance conductors are involved, you need to determine a size equal to the largest service-entrance conductor by calculating the largest sum of the areas of conductors that correspond to each other in each set. However, if no service-entrance conductors are involved, then you have to calculate the largest sum of the areas of the service-entrance conductors that would be needed to service the electrical load involved. NEC 250.70 lists the specific means required for connecting grounding electrodes to a grounding conductor as follows:

- Exothermic welding

- Listed lugs or pressure connectors

- Approved ground clamps that are listed for the grounding conductor materials and are rated for direct soil burial or concrete encasement if they are used on pipes, rods, or other buried electrodes

Next, you have to consider the type of grounding electrode application you will be using and size the grounding electrode conductor accordingly. For example, if you are connecting a grounding electrode conductor to a rod, pipe, or plate, then the part of the conductor that is the solitary connection to the grounding electrode does not have to be any larger than 6 AWG copper or 4 AWG aluminum wire. For connections to concrete-encased electrodes, the portion of the conductor that is the lone connection to the grounding electrode is not required to be larger than 4 AWG copper wire. If you plan to connect the grounding electrode conductor to a ground ring, then the segment of the conductor that is the sole connection to the grounding electrode does not have to be any larger than the conductor that is used in the grounding ring.

Remember one thing when dealing with grounding electrode conductors: any connections you make have to not only be accessible, but must also create an effective and permanent grounding path.

The water pipe system in a building is not allowed to be the sole grounding source. A supplemental electrode, such as a ground rod, must be installed if the water piping system would otherwise be the only source of grounding.

GROUNDING ELECTRODE CONDUCTOR SAFETY

Have you ever started to connect or reconnect a grounding electrode conductor to the ground rod and seen it spark? Maybe you have been disconnecting a grounding electrode from a water pipe and been shocked. I have heard electricians attribute this to "phantom" current, phase imbalance, and even "bad" ground rods or condensation. The shocking truth is simply that grounding electrode conductors regularly carry current. This doesn't make sense to some people based on their interpretation, or rather misinterpretation, of NEC 250.2, as well as the theory of "least resistance."

NEC 250.2 describes an effective ground fault current path as an intentionally constructed, permanent, low-impedance electrically conductive path designed and intended to carry current under ground fault conditions from the point of a ground fault to the electrical supply source. The use of the word "ground" in the definition is often misconstrued to imply that the grounding electrode conductor is part of the fault-clearing path, and that any current will only exist temporarily until an overcurrent protective device opens the circuit.

Furthermore, the presence of current in a grounding electrode conductor can be the result of an open neutral and current resistance. In a standard residential electrical system, the neutral conductor carries the imbalance current of the system. An open neutral in the neighbor's house can allow the imbalance current from the neighboring building to follow a path back through a water pipe common to both buildings. From there it will flow up through the grounding electrode conductor of the adjacent building (Figure 5.7).

The first safety step involving grounding electrode conductors is to find out if there is an open neutral in your system. This is done by measuring a potential difference in the various loads in the building. You can use your ammeter to measure for current in the grounding electrode conductor before you open up that connection. If you discover a current, the next thing you must determine is in which direction the current is flowing. Is the current going "down" into the ground from the building

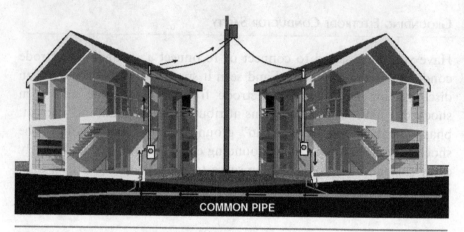

COMMON PIPE

Figure 5.7 An open neutral exists in the house on the right. The imbalance current from the neighboring home flows back through the common water main and up through the grounding electrode conductor of the building on the left.

you are working on or is it coming up through the grounding electrode conductor in your building and returning back to the source by means of your neutral?

Since using an ammeter on the conductor will only indicate the presence of current and not the direction of the current flow, you will need to apply Kirchoff's Law to determine current path. Kirchoff's Law uses the premise that all currents entering a connection are equal to the currents leaving a connection, which means that all currents must balance. Here is an example of Kirchoff's Law.

You will be working on a residential single-phase, 120/240 V service. Never assume that a grounding electrode conductor is dead. First you measure 11 A in the black conductor at the main service panel, and then 5 A in the red conductor. On a single-phase service, the neutral current is the difference between the two legs of the transformer, which comes out to 6 A. To trace the current flow, if you measure 6 A in the grounding electrode conductor and 0 A in the neutral service entrance conductor, you know that the neutral is open. This means the current is flowing from the building you are working on into an alternate return path, in this case the grounding electrode. If there is no current in one of the grounding electrode conductors, this doesn't

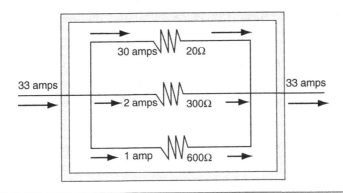

Figure 5.8   Current returns through all paths, not just the path of least resistance.

mean there is no grounding electrode current flowing somewhere in the system. Test for current in all grounding electrode connection points individually.

The other factor that affects current in a grounding electrode conductor is the theory of the path of least resistance. All of us have heard the expression that electrical current will follow the path of least resistance, but what does that really mean? Current will always attempt to flow back to the electrical source. If there are multiple paths back to the source, current will flow through all the paths to reach its destination, with the majority of current flowing through the path of least resistance. But the lower amount of current is still electricity that can shock and injury you (Figure 5.8).

GROUNDING AC SYSTEMS

Alternating-current systems are required to be grounded per NEC 250.20. For systems that are less than 50 V, you need to ground installations that are supplied by transformers that exceed 150 V to ground, or if the transformer supply is ungrounded or installed as overhead conductors outside of a building. If the systems have a supply between 50 and 1000 V, you will have to ground them in one of the following ways:

- So that the maximum voltage to ground on the ungrounded conductors is not any greater than 150 V

- The neutral of a three-phase, four-wire wye system is used as a circuit conductor

- Or, for a three-phase, four-wire delta, the midpoint of one phase winding is used as a circuit conductor

There are a number of scenarios where you can ground AC systems, but you don't have to. This would be for systems that range from 50 to 1000 V with ground detectors and which fall into one of the following categories:

1. An electrical system that is exclusively used to supply an industrial furnace that is used for melting, refining, or tempering.

2. Separately derived systems that are only used for rectifiers that only supply adjustable-speed industrial drives. A rectifier is a device that converts alternating current to DC or to current with only positive value. This process is referred to as rectification. Rectifiers can be made of solid state diodes, vacuum tube diodes, mercury arc valves, and other similar components.

3. Separately derived systems that are supplied by transformers with a primary voltage that is less than 1000 V and which are only used for control circuits will only be accessible to qualified persons, have control power continuity, and include ground detectors on the control system.

When grounding an AC service, you need to install a grounding electrode conductor and connect it to a grounded service conductor at each service. Some circuits listed in NEC 250.22 are not permitted to be grounded. That's right, you are NOT allowed to ground circuits in installations such as health care facility anesthetizing locations, induction rooms, or circuits that supply medical equipment that uses 150 V or more, such as portable X-ray machines. Do not ground secondary light system circuits either. You are also prohibited from grounding circuits for electric cranes that are used over Class III location combustible fibers, or for equipment within electrolytic cell working zones.

EQUIPMENT GROUNDING

Equipment that is fastened in place or connected with fixed, permanent wiring methods must have the exposed non-current carrying metal parts grounded based on NEC 250.110. The types of equipment that must be grounded regardless of the voltage involved are listed below:

- Switchboard frames and structures, unless it is a DC two-wire switchboard that is already effectively insulated from ground

- Pipe organs

- Motor frames and motor controller enclosures

- Elevators and cranes

- Commercial garages, theaters, and motion picture studio electrical equipment, except for pendant lamp holders with circuits of 150 V to ground or less (motion picture projection equipment must also be grounded)

- Electric signs

- Power-limited remote-control, signaling and fire alarm circuits that have system grounding requirements provided in NEC 250.112 Part II or Part IV

- Light fixtures

- Permanently mounted skid equipment

- Motor-operated water pumps

- Metal well casings

There are 14 types of EGCs listed in NEC 250.118 that are approved for use to enclose the conductors of power supply circuits or to run with them. These can be used individually or in combination and are as follows:

- Solid or stranded copper, aluminum, or copper-clad aluminum conductors which may be insulated, covered, or bare and in the form of a wire or busbar of any shape

- Rigid metal conduit

- Intermediate metal conduit

- Electrical metal tubing

- Flexible metal conduits that meet one of the following criteria: are terminated in fittings that are approved for grounding; circuit conductors in conduit that are protected by 20 A or less OCPDs; have a combined length of flexible conduit materials in the same ground return path that does not exceed 6 feet; will have an EGC installed

■ Flexible metallic tubing that is listed for grounding and has conductors in conduit that are protected by 20 A or less OCPDs as well as a combined length of flexible and liquid-tight conduit in the same ground return path that does not exceed 6 feet

■ Listed liquid-tight flexible metal conduit that meets the following standards: is terminated in fittings that are approved for grounding; circuit conductors that are ⅜-½ inch (#12 to #16) in conduit that are protected by 20 A or less OCPDs; circuit conductors that are ¾ to 1 ¼ inch (#21 to #35) in conduit that are protected by OCPDs that are rated at 60 A or less and are not run with flexible metal or liquid-tight conduit that is ⅜-½ inch (#12 to #16) in the grounding path; the total combined length of the flexible and liquid-tight conduits in the same ground path does not exceed 6 feet; an EGC is installed

■ The copper sheath of metal sheathed, mineral-insulated cable

■ Type AC cable armor

■ Type MC cable that is identified and listed for grounding, as long as the metal sheath and grounding conductor are of interlocked metal tape type MC cable or are smooth or corrugated tube type MC cable

■ Cable trays

■ Cablebus framework

■ Surface metal raceways that are listed for grounding

■ Other listed metal raceways and auxiliary gutters

**Cable assemblies and flexible cords as outlined in NEC 250.138.

The standards for sizing EGCs are provided in NEC 250.122. For the general rules for sizing, refer to NEC Table 250.122.

If you have to increase the size of ungrounded conductors then you need to bump up the size of the EGCs proportionally to the circular mil area of the ungrounded conductors.

For multiple circuits that are run with a single EGC in the same raceway, you need to be sure to size the EGC for the largest overcurrent device that protects the raceway conductors. Motor circuits with overcurrent devices that consist of an instantaneous trip circuit or a motor short-circuit protector can have an EGC that is sized based on the rating of the motor overload protection device as long as you don't use a size that is less than what is listed in NEC Table 250.122.

If the equipment in a system has ground-fault protection installed, each parallel EGC that is in a multi-conductor cable should be sized based on NEC Table 250.112 based on the trip rating of the ground-fault protection. Additionally, the ground-fault protection needs to be installed in a manner so that only qualified people can maintain or service the installation. The ground-fault protection equipment must also be set to trip at no more than the amperage of any single ungrounded conductor of one of the cables in parallel, and it must be rated for use in protecting the EGC.

GROUNDED NEUTRAL CONDUCTORS

Keeping the normal current that flows across a neutral conductor on the path it was intended to follow is an important aspect of safety and noise over the grounded paths, including the EGCs of a system. NEC Section 250.142(B), Exceptions 1 through 4, provide restrictive conditions for using the grounded (neutral) conductor for grounding on the load side of the service disconnect as follows:

- On the supply-side of equipment you can ground non-current carrying metal parts of equipment, raceways, and other enclosures with a grounded circuit conductor only at these locations:
  - On the supply side, or within the enclosure of, the AC service-disconnecting means
  - On the supply side or within the enclosure of the main disconnecting means for separate buildings. You need to refer to NEC 250.32(B) as a cross reference for the standards for separate buildings which require that the EGCs be run with supply conductors and be connected to the building structures or disconnecting means and to the grounding electrodes

■ On the supply side, or within the enclosure of the main disconnecting means or overcurrent devices of a separately derived system as permitted by NEC 250.30(A)(1)

■ On the load-side of equipment of the service disconnecting means or the load side of a separately derived system disconnecting means or the overcurrent devices for a separately derived system that do not have a main disconnecting means you can only use a grounded circuit conductor for grounding the non-current carrying metal parts of equipment as permitted in 250.30(A)(1) and 250.32(B)

GROUNDING HIGH VOLTAGE SYSTEMS

When grounding high voltage systems that are 1 kV or higher, you need to follow the standards in NEC Part X. You can use a system neutral that is derived from a grounding transformer to ground high voltage systems. A single point grounded or multi-grounded neutral can be used for solidly grounded neutral systems and the neutral conductor needs to have a minimum insulation level of 600 V. The exceptions would be for the neutral conductors in overhead installations, service entrances, and direct buried portions of feeders, in which case the neutral conductors can be bare copper (Figure 5.9).

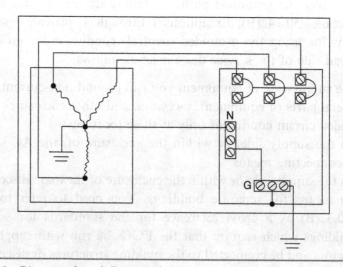

Figure 5.9 Diagram of a solidly grounded system.

The ampacity of the high voltage neutral conductor has to be sufficient to carry the load and not less than 33⅓% of the phase conductor amperage unless it is for an industrial or commercial installation. For industrial and commercial premises, you can size the neutral conductor at no less than 20% of the phase conductor amperage as long as it is done with engineering supervision. If you intended to use a single point grounded system, you need to refer to NEC 250.184(B) 1-8 for the standard requirements. Portable and mobile high voltage equipment must be supplied from a system that has its neutral grounded through an impedance. If you are connecting to a delta-connected high voltage system then a system neutral needs to be derived. Finally, the voltage that is developed between the portable or mobile equipment and ground by the flow of the maximum ground-fault current cannot be greater than 100 V. Grounding conductors that are not an integral part of a cable assembly cannot be smaller than 6 AWG copper or 4 AWG aluminum and the metal, non-current carrying parts of the mobile or portable equipment, enclosures, or fencing must be grounded.

Let's look at an example of this code's application. Assume you are going to layout the grounding system for an industrial piping plant with steel buildings and equipment that is mounted on foundations that are not under cover. The foundations are going to have rebar reinforcement and the equipment needs to be attached to a grounding loop that has been routed throughout the plant. You need to determine if the foundation rebar is required to be attached to the grounding system or grounded at any point at all. If the foundations meet the description in NEC 250.52 (A)(3) for concrete-encased electrodes, the foundations are required to be part of the grounding electrode system at each building or structure.

The NEC only requires an earth resistance value of 25 ohms for single rod, pipe or plate electrode grounding electrode systems. Additionally, installations must comply with the overall performance objectives which can mean that testing of the grounding electrode system is needed, particularly in the case of connecting a new installation to an existing grounding electrode system that can't be visibly inspected. You also need to consider that an electrical system must be able to be maintained during its operational life in order to protect people and property from electrical hazards.

Artificial earth

Once you leave the service, the role of earth in the grounding system is no more. The EGC is what most of us recognize as the green "ground wire" that is run with electrical circuits. This conductor connects all metal conduits and equipment enclosures to the service ground point. The EGC inside a building serves the same purpose as the earth outside, to provide a low-impedance return path for fault or leaking currents in the event of insulation failure or inadvertent contact of an energized conductor in an enclosure.

The size of the EGC for each circuit is also specified, and is based on the rating of the fuse or circuit breaker protecting the circuit. If proper bonding connections are used to maintain electrical continuity, then metal conduits can act as the EGC without the need to provide an additional conductor in the circuit. Just remember that if the EGC, regardless of whether it is the conduit itself or contained within the conduit along with the circuit conductors, creates a physical separation between conductors and increases the impedance of the current path while reducing the effectiveness of the ground. An EGC must be provided for every circuit.

OSHA Grounding Requirements

OSHA 1910.304(g) requires systems that supply buildings with wiring to be grounded and outlines the means of grounding to be used. For example, OSHA requires all AC circuits that are less than 50 V to be grounded if they are installed as overhead conductors outside of buildings. These circuits must also be grounded if they are supplied by transformers where the primary supply system is either ungrounded or exceeds 150 V to ground. All AC systems between 50 and 1000 V must be grounded. The conductor for AC wiring systems is required to be grounded as follows:

- One conductor of a single-phase, two-wire system must be grounded

- The neutral conductor of a single-phase, three-wire system must be grounded

- The common conductor of a multiphase system that has one wire common to all phases must be grounded

- One phase conductor of a multiphase system, where one phase is grounded, requires grounding

- The neutral conductor of a multiphase system that uses one phase as a neutral conductor needs to be grounded

All three-wire DC systems need to have a grounded neutral conductor, and any two-wire DC systems that operate from 50 to 300 V between conductors must be grounded.

GROUNDING IN GROUNDED SYSTEMS

The NEC requires the grounding (earthing) of the system windings to limit the voltage imposed on the system from lightning, unintentional contact with higher-voltage lines, or line surges. Another function of this earthing is to "stabilize the voltage to earth during normal operation" by providing a common reference point. The code also requires the grounding of metal parts of electrical equipment in or on a building or structure. NEC 250.24 requires that this ground connection be made between the line side of the service equipment and the supply source, such as a utility transformer. This grounding is accomplished by electrically connecting the building or structure disconnecting means with a grounding electrode conductor to a grounding electrode.

Grounding (earthing) in grounded systems has limitations. For example, grounding of electrical equipment doesn't serve the purpose of "providing a low-impedance fault-current path to clear ground faults." In fact, the code prohibits the use of the earth as the sole return path because it's a poor conductor of current at voltage levels below 600 V. Grounding the metal parts of electrical equipment doesn't protect electrical or electronic equipment from lightning-induced voltage transients or high-frequency voltage impulses on the circuit conductors inside the building or structure. It also does not protect equipment within a structure from transients generated from other equipment in the same structure.

Any work involving adding sub-panels, upgrading the electrical service, changing the water service, or re-piping a structure requires upgrading the grounding and bonding of the electrical service.

OBJECTIONABLE CURRENT

Simply put, there are good kinds of current and objectionable types of current. NEC 250.6 provides requirements for preventing the flow of objectionable current over grounding conductors. What it does not spell out clearly is the level of current that would be deemed as objectionable in any given situation. However, when you combine the definitions of grounding found in NEC 100 and NEC 250.2 you get a clear idea of what makes current objectionable and how to prevent it. Grounding conductors are not meant to be used as circuit conductors for functions other than those specifically laid out in NEC 250.4. In most electrical installations current will flow through capacitive coupling. Any potential or associated shock or fire hazards for an installation helps to clarify what levels of current are unsafe or "objectionable." Essentially, objectionable current is simply any level of current in an electrical installation that would pose an electric shock or fire hazard or hinder the ability of the grounding system to perform its intended functions. An example of an objectionable current would be a rise in potential on exposed metal parts that are not designed or meant to be energized, because this kind of situation could produce an electric shock or result in a fire hazard. Another scenario would be excessive current that would interfere with the proper operation of electrical or electronic equipment. NEC 250.6 requires that materials and equipment be installed and arranged in a way that prevents objectionable current from flowing over the grounding conductors or grounding paths.

However, if the use of multiple grounding conductors would actually induce or allow objectionable current, then you are allowed to make several alterations as long as there is an effective ground-fault current path and a path for fault current is provided. These safe adjustments include the following steps:

- You can disconnect one or more grounding connections, just not all of them

- You are allowed to change the locations of grounding conductors

- You could take other suitable corrective actions

- You could even interrupt the continuity of the grounding conductor or the conductive pathway interconnecting the grounding conductors

Bonding

Electrical bonding is the practice of intentionally electrically connecting all metallic non-current carrying items, such as pipes, in a building to form a conductive path and protect against electric shock. The result is that if there is a breach in any of the electrical insulation in a system, all of the metal objects in the room will have the same electrical potential. This way anyone in the room will not touch two objects with significantly different potentials. Even if the grounding connection to earth fails, people will still be protected from dangerous potential differences. Bonding metal parts to each other and then bonding the metal parts to the system provides the process required for over-current protection devices to do their job.

Bonding must consist of a continuous bond jumper installed at the water heater between the hot and cold lines, and, if applicable, gas lines.

Bonding jumpers are used to facilitate bonding. Since bonding jumpers are used in several ways, they are referred to by different names. The main bonding jumper is installed at the service and you will only have one. NEC Article 100 defines a main bonding jumper as a connection between a grounded circuit conductor and the EGC at the electrical service. Based on NEC 250.24, you can install a main bonding jumper at the building service depending on whether an EGC is run with the feeder conductors. System bonding jumpers are installed at separately derived systems and there is one for each separately derived system that is utilized (Figure 5.10).

Both of these types of bonding jumpers do the same thing. They provide an effective ground fault current path from your equipment enclosures and raceways to the electrical source. Equipment bonding jumpers are used to tie equipment together in order to keep voltage from building up in equipment and creating a difference in potential between various pieces of equipment. For example, if you were bonding two metal raceways together, you would use an equipment bonding jumper anywhere there was a break in the metal conduit run. An equipment bonding jumper is not required for receptacles attached to listed exposed work covers when certain conditions are met. These conditions are that

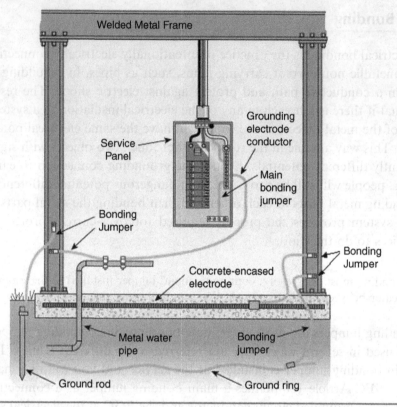

Figure 5.10 Types and locations of bonding jumpers.

the receptacle is attached to the cover with two permanent rivets, or has a threaded or screwed locking means, and when the cover mounting holes are located on a flat non-raised portion of the cover. This is because exposed work covers with two fasteners that are used to attach the receptacle to the cover are considered a suitable bonding means.

A circuit bonding jumper ties together the various conductors of a circuit and it must have the ability to carry the same, or greater, current as the circuit conductors it is connecting. Based on NEC 250.4(A), in order to establish an effective ground-fault current path, those same non-conductive current-carrying materials must be bonded together and to the electrical supply source. Additionally, any electrically conductive materials that are likely to become energized must be bonded in the same manner.

If the main water service piping to the house is metallic, the bonding must be established within 5 feet of where the water piping enters the building.

Ungrounded systems

The general requirements for grounding electrical equipment in ungrounded systems differ in purpose from those for grounded systems. Without system grounding there is no stabilization of the system voltage to earth. This is why you need to limit the voltage (at the equipment level rather than at the system level) that would be imposed by lightning, unintentional contact with higher-voltage lines, or line surges.

Whether your system is grounded or ungrounded, you must bond enclosures and equipment together. In ungrounded systems, bonding of electrical equipment per NEC 250.4(B)(2) serves a purpose similar to that set forth for bonding electrical equipment in grounded systems per NEC 250.4(A)(3). The difference here is you are bonding the equipment parts of an ungrounded system to each other, rather than to each other and the source.

One consequence of this arrangement is the equipment bonding path must be capable of carrying the maximum fault current likely to be imposed on it. Remember, the bonding system must be able to remove dangerous voltage from a second ground fault. The same difference and consequence applies to the bonding of electrically conductive materials and other equipment in ungrounded systems set out in NEC 250.4(B)(3) versus those in grounded systems per NEC 250.4(A)(4). The requirement that all grounding electrodes present at each served building must be bonded together to create a grounding electrode system is the focus of NEC 250.50.

Any of the non-current carrying metal parts of the following types of equipment must be effectively bonded together:

- Cable trays or cablebus framework

- Service raceways or cable armor

- Auxiliary gutters

- Service enclosures that house service conductors such as meter fittings or boxes that are inserted in the service armor or raceways

- Any metallic raceway or armor that encloses a grounding electrode conductor

You must bond at each end of a raceway as well as to any intervening raceways, boxes, or other enclosures anywhere between the service equipment and the grounding electrode.

NEC 250.94 refers to bonding "other" systems by providing an accessible location outside of enclosures for connecting intersystems. It includes a requirement for a well-defined, dedicated location for terminating bonding and grounding conductors on a specific set of terminals or a bonding bar. The termination must have adequate capacity to handle multiple communication systems, such as satellite, CATV, and telecommunication at the premises, and at least three terminals are required. Specifying the termination locations for the intersystem bonding termination is the key part of this revision. The termination means must be secured electrically and mechanically to the premise meter enclosure that is located at either the service equipment enclosure or at the grounding electrode conductor.

Types of Bonding Jumpers

NEC 250.102 provides standards for equipment bonding jumpers. This type of bonding jumper must be copper or some other kind of corrosion-resistant material and can be a bus, screw, wire, or similar form of conductor. Equipment bonding jumpers that are installed on the supply side of a service cannot be any smaller than the sizes for grounding electrode conductors that are listed in NEC Table 250.66. Additional requirements are also applied. For example, if the service-entrance phase conductors are bigger than 1100 kcmil copper, or 1750 kcmil aluminum, then the equipment bonding jumper must have an area that is at least 12½% of the area size of the largest phase conductor. However, if the phase conductors and the bonding jumper are made of different materials, the minimum size of the bonding jumper needs to be based on the "assumed use" of phase conductors. This means you would first assume that the conductors were made of the same materials, even though they are not, and with an equal amperage of the installed phase conductors, and then you would determine the sizing based on that premise. For service-entrance conductors that are installed parallel in two or more raceways, the equipment bonding jumpers must also be run in parallel if they are routed with raceways or cables. In this kind of an installation, the bonding jumper size for each of the raceways or cables would be based on the size of the service-entrance conductors in each of the cables or raceways.

Equipment bonding jumpers that are installed on the load side of service overcurrent protection devices need to have a minimum size that is based on the requirements of NEC Table 250.122. However, these bonding jumpers cannot ever be any smaller than 14 AWG, and they don't have to be any larger than the largest ungrounded circuit conductors that supply the equipment (Figure 5.11).

Two of the most typical means of bonding are to pipes and metal structures, and bonding jumper methods for these are covered in NEC 250.104. Metal water pipes need to be grounded to one of the following:

- The service equipment enclosure

- The grounded conductor at the electrical service

- The grounding electrode conductor if it is a sufficient size

According to Section 250.104(A) you need to refer to Table 250.66 to determine the required sizes for these bonding jumpers. For example, if you needed to bond the interior metal water piping of a building with an electric service that is supplied with 3/0 copper, you would use a

Minimum Copper AWG	Minimum Aluminum or Copper-Clad Aluminum AWG	Amperage Setting/Rating of Automatic Overcurrent Device in the Circuit **Ahead** of the Equipment, Conduit, etc.
14	12	15 amps
12	10	20 amps
10	8	30 amps
10	8	40 amps
10	8	60 amps
8	6	100 amps
6	4	200 amps
4	2	300 amps
3	1	400 amps
2	1/0	500 amps
1	2/0	600 amps
1/0	3/0	800 amps
2/0	4/0	1000 amps
3/0	250	1200 amps
4/0	350	1600 amps
250	400	2000 amps
350	600	2500 amps
400	600	3000 amps
500	800	4000 amps
700	1200	5000 amps
800	1200	6000 amps

Figure 5.11 The size for equipment grounding conductors that ground raceways or equipment must meet these minimum requirements.

4 AWG copper bonding jumper. However, NEC 250.104(A) describes multiple occupancy building bonding requirements. Let's look at an example of how to apply these requirements.

Assume that a service is supplied with two parallel sets of 500 kcmil. Based on this section and its reference to Table 250.66, it would require a 2/0 AWG copper bonding jumper. Now you might ask yourself, if the cold water is bonded at the water service, why does the hot water piping require such a large bonding jumper? First, look at the general requirement for bonding metal water piping systems that is contained in 250.104(A). This describes that any metal piping system used for water, whether it is for a domestic supply or other use, is treated as a metal water piping system and is required to be bonded to the electrical services and systems that are in or on the same building or area of a building.

If the electrical system does not contain equipment grounds, then the water or gas piping system must be bonded externally with a bonding jumper.

If it is determined that the piping system is electrically continuous, a single connection to any point on the piping system will comply with this requirement. The bonding conductor or jumper is sized using Table 250.66. Next, if there is some dielectric separating the hot water pipes from the cold-water piping, a bonding jumper of the same size as the bonding conductor run from the service equipment or separately derived system is required. This ensures that all of the metal water piping system is bonded using a fully sized bonding conductor or jumper (Figure 5.12).

By looking back at NEC Table 250.66 to pick the bonding conductors and bonding jumpers, you will see that this standard is providing a worst-case scenario approach. This ensures that there is a sufficient path for ground fault current in the event that the metal water piping becomes energized because the electrical system fails somewhere. In addition to supplying this ground fault current path, bonding of the metal water piping system serves as an equipotential connection to reduce the likelihood of electric shock hazards at interfaces where the

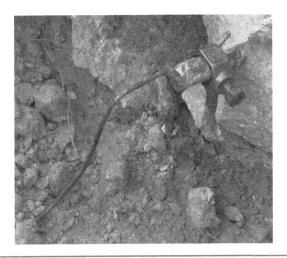

Figure 5.12   A bonding jumper attached to rebar which is encased in concrete.

conductive surfaces of equipment supplied by the electrical system and by the water system are both present.

There are two vital reasons for grounding and bonding. One is to protect people who come in contact with energized metal parts due to a ground-fault, and the other is to ensure that the fault is quickly resolved before a fire develops (Figure 5.00).

GROUNDING AND BONDING FAST FACTS

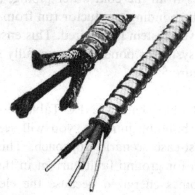

The following AC systems **must be grounded**:

AC systems less than 50 volts
AC systems from 50 to 1000 volts
AC systems over 1kV
Separately derived systems

Circuits that **should NOT be grounded**, due to their designated use:

- Circuits for electric cranes used in Class III locations because of the combustible fibers which are easily ignited by an sparking or acing devices

- Circuits in health care facilities for equipment such as anesthesia or in operating rooms

- Secondary circuits for lighting systems

Grounding Electrode Conductor Use

A grounding electrode conductor needs to be installed to bond and ground the service equipment terminal neutral bus to the grounding electrode system

Generator Bonding Jumper: A generator bonding jumper collets all of the fault current in amps that can be gathered at the bonding connection and transfers it, allowing the current to flow through the windings of a generator and balancer set.

Figure 5.00 Know your grounding and bonding facts.

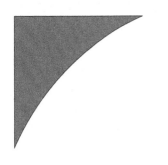

Chapter 6

Safety Grounding Principals

Chapter Outline

Think of electrical current as energy that flows in a loop. If you have a wire carrying current from one device to another, there must be a second wire for the current to get back. If the loop is interrupted or broken, the current will try to continue to move through any conductive material, including your body. We have already reviewed the importance of matching your experience, training, and technical skill with the task as hand.

123

Doi: 10.1016/B978-1-85617-654-5.00006-6

The safest work scenario is one that involves the absence of electrical current, but as an electrician that doesn't happen. Even in new construction projects, at some point appliances and equipment will eventually have to be connected to power. To reduce the potential for electric shock, safety grounding techniques are used.

Safety grounds

Many terms used in the electrical industry are very similar or can have several meanings or methods of application. Such is the case with safety grounds that cover a broad range of applications. The most common safety ground technique is illustrated with the three-prong receptacle.

The NEC requires all new 120-volt household receptacle outlets, for general-purpose use, to be both grounded and polarized. A correctly installed receptacle should always be vertical with the ground pin beneath the two parallel blade slots. For this reason NEMA adopted the U.S. standard socket configuration that includes a slot for a center-line, rounded pin connected to a safety ground to facilitate the ground and two blade-shaped slots of uniform but differing sizes to prevent ungrounded (two-wire) devices from being incorrectly connected. Additionally, the NEC requires 240-volt center tapped single-phase receptacles with two slots for "hot" current and a neutral center tap.

As an electrician, you may be contacted by homeowners who are purchasing or remodeling an older property with fuses and wish to convert to circuit breakers to meet current code requirements. These customers may not realize that they cannot simply change out their two-prong outlets with three-prong receptacles without also running new code compliant wiring. Often this is because people have made do by rigging three-prong adapters to two-prong outlets or extension cords without understanding the need for establishing a safety ground (Figure 6.1).

In the case of extension cords, the metal connector of these adapters does not come in contact with a metal grounding source, consequently the need behind generating a safety ground is not met, creating the possibility of electrical shock. It becomes your responsibility to educate these

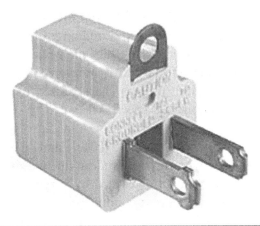

Figure 6.1 Three-prong adapters do not take the place of code-compliant outlets with a safety ground.

customers on the requirements and mechanics of safety grounds and the wiring necessary to comply with creating the ground system. NEC Section 406.3 stipulates that receptacle outlets must be of the grounding type, with a minimum wire size of 14 AWG (CU) and 12 AWG (AL) for 15-amp circuits and 12 AWG 10 AWG for a 20-amp circuit.

NEC 406.3(D)(3) permits the use of grounding-type receptacles in non-grounded wiring if a GFCI is used for protection of the outlet.

ISOLATED GROUND

Electronic equipment, such as computer servers and other voltage or noise sensitive systems, requires regulation of the supply to these loads that is improved by using an isolated ground. Isolated ground receptacles, which are bright orange with a triangle marked on the face, are used. Basically, these receptacles have a separate "green wire" equipment ground, and the wire goes back directly to the circuit breaker panel, without being connected to anything else. If you use an isolated ground receptacle down line from the panel board, the isolated ground conductor is not connected to the conduit or panel enclosure, rather to the ground conductor of the supply feeder. In this case, the conduit acts as the safety ground, but a separate conductor can also be used for the safety ground as described in NEC 274.

Isolated ground receptacles are installed to protect electronic equipment from the electrical noise generated in a building. Electronic noise is an unwanted signal characteristic of all electronic circuits that comes from many different electronic effects and is measured in watts of power. Electronic noise is a random process characterized by properties such as its variance, distribution, and spectral density.

Types of noise include shot, thermal, flicker, and burst signals. Shot noise in electronic devices consists of random fluctuations of the electric current in an electrical conductor, caused by varying electron charges. Thermal noise is generated across conductors as free charges generate kinetic energy from their motion, resulting in kinetic noise. Flicker noise, also known as $1/f$ noise, is a signal variation present in almost all electronic devices. Burst noise consists of sudden transitions between two or more levels, as high as several hundred millivolts, which occurs at random and unpredictable times.

To protect against damage to sensitive electronics, an isolated ground consists of a black "hot" wire that goes to the brass or copper screw in an outlet which is connected to the smaller right side receptacle slot. The white neutral wire goes to the silver or chrome screw that is connected to the larger left side slot and the bare, safety ground wire goes to the green screw for the separate ground path.

SINGLE-POINT GROUNDING

NEC 250 states that a single-point grounding system is one in which all electrical references to ground come to a single point in the building before attaching to the earth. Use an isolated ground, neutral conductor or safety ground connected to an equipment cabinet and come to a single-point at the main distribution panel and then connect to the earth grounding system associated with the structure. All system grounds terminate to this single connecting point (Figure 6.2).

This creates a condition where each component and external source is effectively bonded to a single point, which is then effectively bonded to the building or external ground system. In this way, all of the equipment, including power, telephone, cable TV, etc., is bonded to a single

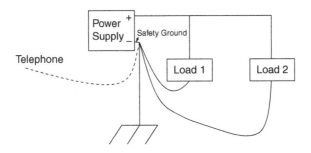

Figure 6.2   An example of single point grounding with safety ground.

common ground point. Therefore, little current will flow between these systems, allowing essentially no difference of potential between the electrical components inside the building surges such as lightning activity. In the event of a lightning strike, inductively coupled energy would be coupled into the building structure or circuit conductors within the facility.

> The NEC prohibits the use of mounting hardware to double as a safety ground because it seeks to have a person physically undo the safety ground rather than "accidentally" undo the safety ground during normal servicing operations.

THREE-PHASE DISTRIBUTION GROUND

Three-phase systems are used to distribute high power to buildings and are suitable for driving powerful electric motor equipment. The wiring is designed so that the power drawn from each phase is equal. This is accomplished by connecting all high-power loads to all three phases and distributing all of the smaller loads to those three phases.

Three-phase power has three "hot" wires, 120° out of phase with each other. The power comes from the power utility through four current carrying wires: three phase wires and one neutral wire, and the neutral wire is connected to the building ground in the central main distribution panel. If the current is exactly matched in all phases, there is no current flowing in neutral wire.

From the main central distribution panel five wires lead to the subpanels, consisting of four current carrying wires and a neutral wire. In this type of system, the safety ground is a separate wire that also goes to the central grounding bar like a neutral wire. The distinction between a neutral wire and safety ground is that neutral wire carries the difference in current from each phase during normal operations, but the safety ground does not carry any current during normal operations. In this way, the entire safety ground wire exists in the building ground potential during normal operation.

The safety ground wires should be interconnected in a star- or tree-like manner.

Safety grounding jumpers

One method of protecting against contact with electrical current is to utilize safety grounding jumpers which are commonly called safety grounds. Don't confuse safety grounding jumpers with bonding jumpers which are used to form a connection between electrical components such as a grounded circuit conductor (neutral) and an equipment-grounding conductor at a main electrical service. Safety grounding serves to reduce the possibility of electric shock to not only workers, but to equipment as well.

In this application, the safety ground consists of a length of insulated conductive cable with connector clamps on each end. There is no code requirement for the color of the cable insulation, but most often it is yellow, black, or clear. If a circuit accidentally becomes energized, the safety ground will short-circuit and ground the circuit, de-energizing the conductors and protecting personnel. Additionally, safety grounds serve to drain static charge. In order to be effective, a safety ground must be capable of withstanding the thermal and magnetic forces that would travel through the jumper if a circuit became energized. Conductor sizes in the safety ground should be matched with the ultimate short circuit potential (Figure 6.3).

Surges not in excess of 20% asymmetry factor for Withstand and Ultimate Short Circuits							
Copper Grounding cable size	Withstand Rating Symmetrical, kA rms 60 Hz			Ultimate Capacity Symmetrical, kA rms 60 Hz			
	15 cycles (250 ms)	30 cycles (500 ms)	6 cycles (100ms)	15 cycles (500 ms)	30 cycles (500 ms)	60 cycles (1 s)	Continuous current rating rms, 60 Hz
#2	14.5	10	29	18	13	9	200
1/0	21	15	47	29	21	14	250
2/0	27	20	59	37	26	18	300
3/0	36	25	74	47	33	23	350
4/0	43	30	94	59	42	29	400
250 kcmil	54	39	111	70	49	35	450
350 kcmil	74	54	155	98	69	49	550

Figure 6.3 A table listing conductor sizes matched with ultimate capacity and withstand ratings.

Knowing where and when to ground components and cables is as important as knowing that size safety ground that needs to be used. Before you attempt to install safety grounds, take a voltage measurement to verify that the system is de-energized. Don't apply safety grounds if the measurement of insulation resistance can't be done when safety grounds are installed. Safety grounds can be applied on any voltage level system to add additional protection when the system is out of service and conductors are exposed. Qualified personnel should affix safety grounds on systems of 480 V and higher when the circuits are locked and tagged. Lower voltage systems can be safety grounded as needed.

The safety grounds should be installed so that they equalize the voltage on all equipment that is within reach of the person working on the system. Additionally, safety grounds should be applied on both sides of the

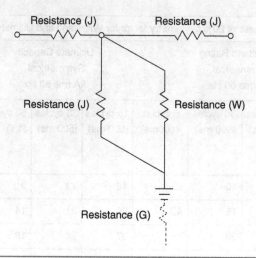

Resistance (J)   Resistance (J)

Resistance (J)   Resistance (W)

Resistance (G)

Figure 6.4   Rj is the safety ground resistance, Rw is the worker resistance, and Rg is the resistance to ground.

work area. In the case of safety grounds, more is better, and the more grounding points you establish, the higher the odds that any accidental current will be eliminated. Remember that you are applying safety grounds to protect against current. This means that applying the safety grounds involves a degree of risk of electric arc, so wear PPE, including a face shield and rubber gloves during the process (Figure 6.4).

Single point ground is the placement of only one safety ground set. In this procedure, the safety grounds are placed as close to the point of work as possible, and when possible, the grounds are placed between the worker and the source of electric energy. Two-point ground is the placement of two safety ground sets. They are usually placed on opposite sides of the work area; that is, one set is placed upstream and one set is placed downstream from the workers.

Let's look at a standard three-wire power distribution system that consists of a hot wire (115 VAC), neutral wire, and safety ground wire. The circuit current is designed to flow from the hot wire, through the load, and through the neutral, but not through the safety ground. By connecting the safety ground to the appliance's enclosure, you are protected from electrocution in the event of a ground fault. However, the neutral and safety ground are common back at the main entrance

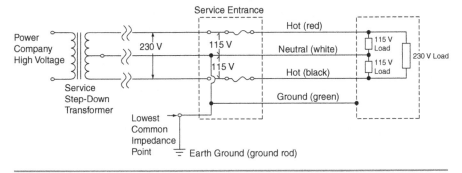

Figure 6.5 A standard AC wiring diagram illustrating safety ground and the lowest common impedance (resistance to current flow) point.

panel. This should be the theoretical single point ground or the lowest common impedance point that equates to the reference ground for the power transformer in the main service power system. Appliances wired for 230 VAC may not use a neutral at all, but the enclosure is typically connected to the safety ground in case of dielectric failure. The reality is that, due to capacitive coupling, some currents flow in the safety ground. Capacitive or electric fields are voltage fields, and capacitive coupling is the transfer of energy between circuits (Figure 6.5).

REMOVING SAFETY GROUNDS

Ideally, safety grounds should be removed using hot sticks, while wearing any necessary personal protection equipment such as rubber gloves, fire retardant clothing, and a face shield. In other words, wear what you would wear to apply the safety grounds when you remove them. Remove each of the phase connections one at a time and remove the ground connection. Remember that the safety grounds need to be removed before the power system is reenergized (Figure 6.6).

EQUIPOTENTIAL GROUND

Safety grounds should be applied in a way to create a zone of equal potential in a high voltage area or area prone to shock hazards. This equipotential zone allows a means for fault current to be bypassed around an area through metal conductors. In this way, a person is protected from shock by the low-resistance metallic conductors of the

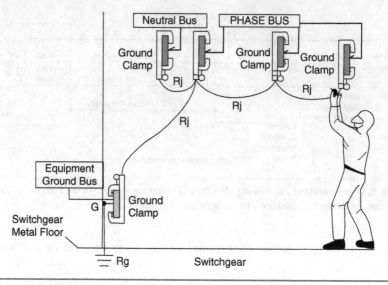

Figure 6.6 Removing safety grounds.

safety ground. For example, what would happen if a worker accidentally contacted the center phase of a safety grounded system under the following conditions: a fault current capacity of 10,000 A, safety ground resistance (Rj) of 0.001 Ω and a worker resistance (Rw) of 500 Ω. The result would be that the worker would receive only about 20 mA of current flow.

OSHA 1910.269 describes several methods that can be employed to protect people from hazardous ground-potential gradients. These include creating equipotential zones and restricted work areas, and insulating equipment. An equipotential zone can be created to protect anyone standing within the zone area from the hazards of step and touch potentials and can be achieved through the installation of a metal mat or interconnected metal grid connected to a grounded object. A grounding grid will equalize the voltage within the grid and produce many alternate paths for electrical energy to find its way back to ground (Figure 6.7).

The distinguishing characteristic of a multipoint grounding grid is that is consists of numerous grounding conductors connected at multiple

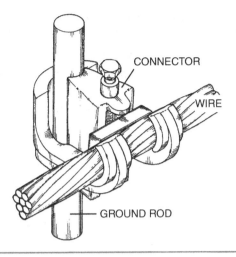

Figure 6.7 Grounding connectors are used to connect grounding conductors.

points in a loose grid configuration. One typical example of the need for an equipotential grid is a pad area around an inground swimming pool—The system of creating an equipotential zone encased in concrete around swimming pools to comply with NEC 680 which requires an equipotential common bonding grid to extend under paved walking surfaces (Figure 6.8).

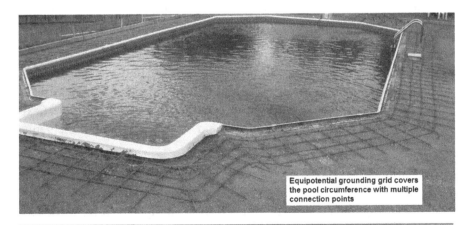

Equipotential grounding grid covers the pool circumference with multiple connection points

Figure 6.8 An equipotential grounding grid protects anyone getting out of the pool from shock hazards because they would have the same electrical charge as the pad.

EQUIPOTENTIAL PLANES AND ANIMAL CONFINEMENT

Unlike equipotential zones, equipotential planes are specifically associated with livestock or animal containment areas. While your grandpa's old barn was primarily made of wood, today's livestock buildings contain extensive networks of electrically conductive materials such as water pipes and feeders, grates, tie-offs, metal mangers, and stall dividers. Often these are accessible by animals housed in the structure. If the electrical equipment or animal enclosures are at a higher electrical potential to earth, this voltage can cause an electric current to flow through an animal if one part of its body is in contact with the equipment and another part is in contact with the earth.

There are a number of terms used in conjunction with equipotential planes and how they are constructed and work. These definitions include:

- *Animal containment areas:* These are areas within a structure that are designated or intended to house or hold animals, such as tie-stalls, milking parlors, and holding areas.

- *Equipotential plane:* A surface that has the same voltage throughout and serves to reduce stray voltage in livestock areas by keeping all animal contact surfaces at the same voltage.

- *Equipment grounding:* Circuits or conducting paths that connect non-current carrying metal parts of equipment, and other metallic surfaces, to the electrical grounding system.

- *Reinforcing rod:* These are steel reinforcing rods that are used to provide tensile strength in concrete and control cracking. Rebar can be used as the conductive medium in concrete to provide exact vertical placement of all the metal and to weld to other structural elements that are embedded in the concrete.

- *Step voltage:* The voltage between two points on the earth's surface separated by a distance of one pace or roughly 3 feet. This voltage can be dangerous if it reaches levels high enough to cause sufficient current flow through a person or animal.

■ *Stray voltage:* Sometimes called "tingle voltage" or "extraneous voltage," this is a low-level voltage, usually less than 10 V, generated in an animal contact area, that is present on metal equipment and can injure livestock. The animal must be able to contact the equipment and the ground or some other equipment at a different voltage before it can be affected.

■ *Touch voltage:* Voltage between a grounded metal structure and a point on the earth's surface separated by a distance equal to the normal maximum reach of a person. This is assumed to be 3 feet for people but can be more or less when dealing with animals. For example, further than 3 feet for a horse but less then 2 feet for a goat.

■ *Voltage ramp:* An area producing a gradual change in voltage from the equipotential plane to the surrounding area created by installing conductive elements.

■ *Wire mesh:* Any 6 by 6-inch square wire grid used to reinforce concrete and provide a conductive gridwork in a concrete floor. Typically the wire sizes used are # 6 AWG to #10 AWG.

An equipotential plane is used to minimize the voltage difference between any metal equipment or structure and the floor. Animals standing or lying on a floor containing a properly installed equipotential plane will have all possible contact points at the same voltage. This will prevent any significant current from flowing through the animal's body, regardless of the neutral to earth voltage. An equipotential plane can be created by installing a bonded network of welded wire mesh or a reinforcing rod in the floor (Figure 6.9).

The bonded network must be electrically connected to the metal structure and equipment and to the system grounding at the electrical service to the building. A series of stanchions or stalls can be interconnected and bonded at one location to meet NEC requirements, and must have at least one exposed connection to the electrical grounding system. This can be done by either extending a reinforcing rod through the top or edge of the concrete near the electrical ground rod or with a copper wire welded to the wire mesh.

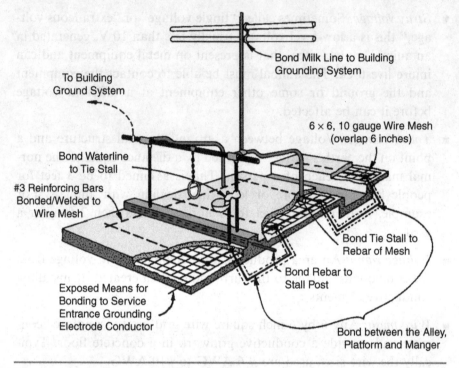

To Building
Ground System

Bond Milk Line to Building
Grounding System

6 × 6, 10 gauge Wire Mesh
(overlap 6 inches)

Bond Waterline
to Tie Stall

#3 Reinforcing Bars
Bonded/Welded to
Wire Mesh

Bond Tie Stall to
Rebar of Mesh

Bond Rebar to
Stall Post

Exposed Means for
Bonding to Service
Entrance Grounding
Electrode Conductor

Bond between the Alley,
Platform and Manger

Figure 6.9   A diagram of a barn's equipotential plane configuration.

Protection Against Varied Voltage

Stray voltage, while not necessarily lethal, can result in a number of behavioral changes in livestock. If you get shocked every time you try to eat or drink, you will hesitate to do it. With livestock such as cows, this reduced feed and water intake can result in reduced milk production and weight loss. NEC 547 specifies that wire mesh or other conductive elements must be installed in the concrete floor of livestock confinement areas and be bonded to the building grounding electrode system to provide an equipotential plane that has a voltage gradient at entrances and exits.

The recommended maximum spacing for #3 (⅜ inch) or larger rebar to control voltage is 12 inches. The reinforcing rod in the base grid should be welded together. The grid should be electrically continuous for the full length and width of the building.

A voltage ramp can be used where the animals can enter or leave an equipotential plane area to allow a gradual increase in step voltage. A voltage gradient is formed by extending the equipotential plane outward and downward at a 45-degree angle. To achieve this, copper-clad ground rods spaced 12 inches apart along the width of the path are driven into the ground at a 45-degree angle to the surface. To complete the plane, these ground rods should be bonded to the equipotential plane before pouring the concrete.

Touch and Step Potential

When a ground fault occurs on a power line, voltage is transferred to the grounded object that is causing the fault in the line. The voltage to this object rises depending on several factors such as the voltage through the power line, the impedance of the faulted conductor, and the impedance to "absolute" ground of the object. For this reason, insulated PPE, such as rubber gloves, should be used to help protect employees who work on or around grounded equipment and conductors from hazardous touch potentials. The PPE needs to be rated for the highest voltage that can be impressed on the grounded objects under fault conditions, not for the full system voltage.

If the object that is causing the fault creates a large impedance, the voltage through it is essentially the phase-to-ground system voltage. Even faults to well-grounded substation structures can pose a serious threat from hazardous voltages depending on the size of the fault current.

There are two types of shock scenarios indicative of power line work that safety grounding guards against. These are "touch potential" and "step potential." Touch potential is the voltage that a person experiences when they "touch" an energized conductor or piece of equipment at the same time that they are in contact with another piece of equipment that produces a different voltage level. Step potential is the difference in the voltage between your feet and a surface beneath your feet that may have a voltage gradient along it.

Here is how these potentials work. When an earth fault current flows back to a transformer neutral it passes through the ground. The resistance of the current path depends on a number of factors including soil composition, resistivity, and moisture. The resistivity of the soil is proportional to the area. This means that the closer the earth path gets to the transformer, the more ground area there is available for the current to pass through. This area reduces by a factor of the distance squared, and as a result the resistance path increases. As the resistance increases it creates a voltage drop across the path of the current.

With step voltage hazards, the voltage gradient across a 1 m span, or typical adult step, of earth defines the earth fault current. This 1 m span is the difference in voltage, based on the voltage distribution curve, between two points that are located at different distances from the electrode. The dissipation of voltage from a grounding electrode or the grounded end of an energized grounded object is known as the "ground potential gradient." The voltage drop associated with this decrease of voltage is referred to as the "ground potential." The further away voltage is from a grounding electrode, the greater the voltage decreases, and this is known as the voltage curve. OSHA 1910.269 describes step potential as the voltage between the feet of a person standing near an energized grounded object. The bottom line is that you can be at risk of injury during a fault just because you are standing near the grounding point (Figure 6.10).

Touch voltage is the difference in voltage during a fault between any two surfaces that could be touched simultaneously. Touch potential is the voltage between an energized object and the feet of a person who might come in contact with the object. This potential is equal to the difference in voltage between the energized object, measured as the base distance of 0 feet, and a point some distance away. Unfortunately, touch potential can be almost equal to the full voltage across the grounded object if the grounded object is located away from where the person is in contact with the object. For example, if a crane is grounded to a system neutral and it contacts an energized line the crane operator (exposed person) would be exposed to a touch potential almost equal to the full fault voltage (Figure 6.11).

An engineering analysis of a power system under fault conditions can help to determine whether or not hazardous step and touch voltages

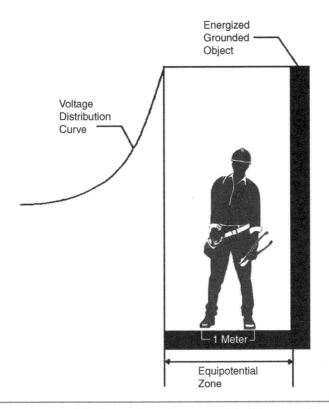

Figure 6.10 Step potential refers to the voltage potential of the ground you stand on.

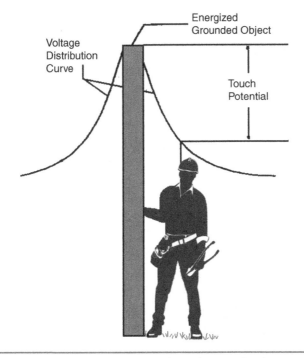

Figure 6.11 Touch potential refers to the voltage that transfers between two surfaces that are touched.

will develop. A touch potential engineering analysis should be done if it is not possible to physically disconnect the system ground or if ground faults are likely to occur. Touch potential measurements don't indicate the ability of a grounding conductor to carry high phase-to-ground fault currents.

Touch potential is measured in volts per ampere of fault current and is then multiplied by the largest anticipated ground fault current value to arrive at the worst-case touch potential for an installation. Use a four-pole ground resistance tester to perform touch potential measurements because it induces a low level fault into the earth close to the installation ground.

For example, if you connect your resistance tester to a system with a maximum fault current of 5000 A and the tester displays a value of 0.100 Ω, you would multiply 5000 A by 0.1, which equals 500 V.

OSHA 1910.269 App C lists several ways of protecting employees from the hazardous ground-potential gradients involved in step and touch potentials, including creating equipotential zones and restricted work areas, and insulating equipment. Creating an equipotential zone will protect a worker standing within it and can be achieved by creating a grounding grid or using a metal mat connected to the grounded object. However, equipotential zones will not protect employees who are standing partially outside the protected area. Bonding conductive objects in the immediate work area can also be used to minimize the potential between the objects and between each object and ground. OSHA notes however that bonding an object outside the work area can increase the touch potential to that object in some cases. OSHA also recommends restricting employees from areas where hazardous step or touch potentials could arise. Workers on the ground in the vicinity of transmission structures should be kept at a safe enough distance away where step voltages are too low to cause injury. The object is to protect unqualified workers who are not directly involved in the operation being performed. Employees should never handle grounded conductors or equipment likely to become energized to hazardous voltages unless the employees are within an equipotential zone or are protected by insulating equipment (Figure 6.00).

STEP and TOUCH
POTENTIALS

OSHA Appendix C to §1910.269 addresses protection from Step and Touch Potentials.

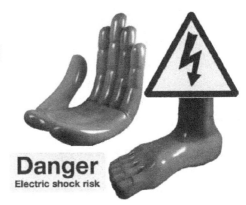

Danger
Electric shock risk

It explains the following hazards:

When a ground fault occurs on a power line, voltage is impressed on whatever grounded object is faulting the line. The voltage to this object will rise, depending on the voltage on the line, the impedance of the faulted conductor, and the impedance to either "true," or "absolute," ground associated with the object.

The term "true ground" literally means that an electrical circuit is connected to the earth (the "ground").

The term absolute ground is misleading because there is a certain amount of resistance to electrical current between all grounding points. No matter how small it is, resistance can always allow electrical voltage to move across it. Consequently, an object can not be "absolutely" grounded.

If an object causes a fault and it has a relatively large impedance, the voltage impressed on it is essentially the phase-to-ground of the system voltage. The degree of the hazard depends upon the size of the fault current and the length of time an object is exposed to the current.

Figure 6.00 OSHA Appendix C to §1910.269 outlines the means for protection from Step and Touch Potentials.

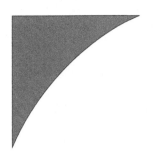

Understanding Arc Flash and Arc Blast Hazards

Chapter 7

Chapter Outline

One of the deadliest hazards any electrician faces is an arc incident. Estimates show that 10 arc-flash incidents occur everyday in the U.S. An electrical arc is a current discharge that is formed when a current jumps a gap in a circuit or between two circuits. An electrical arc can result in a flash or a blast, either of which can be fatal. Let's examine the mechanics of both of these occurrences.

© 2010 Elsevier Inc. All rights reserved.
Doi: 10.1016/B978-1-85617-654-5.00007-8

Electrical faults fall into two categories: bolted faults and arcing faults. A bolted fault occurs when a solidly connected fault path causes high levels of current to flow through the solid connection. The energy in a bolted fault condition is dissipated in the faulted equipment. Arc faults, on the other hand, result in the rapid release of energy caused by arcing between a phase bus bar and another phase bus bar, or a ground or neutral. Several variables affect the generation of an arc flash, including the following:

- The speed of any overcurrent protective devices

- Arc gap spacing

- The size of the enclosure or absence of an enclosure

- The power factor of the fault

- The system voltage

- Whether an arcing fault can sustain itself

- The type of system grounding and bonding present

Arc faults seldom occur in systems with a bus bar voltage lower than 120 V. In the anatomy of an arc fault the air becomes the conductor, and the fault itself is caused by a conductive path or a failure such as broken insulation. One of the major characteristics of an arc fault is the progression of the fault and the effect on other energized parts of the system caused by the buildup of ionized matter within the arc. For example, a line-to-ground arcing fault can quickly become a three-phase arcing fault because the ionized gas produced envelops the other energized part of the equipment.

Initially a precipitating short creates a flash of unconfined electricity and the arc fault is sustained by any added energy from surrounding equipment, as well as the resulting plasma that is highly conductive. This plasma will continue to conduct the available energy present, which is only limited by the impedance of the arc. The intense heat can reach temperatures of 35,000°F, which is about four times the temperature of the sun. What happens next is just as scary. This intense heat rapidly melts or vaporizes the copper components of the

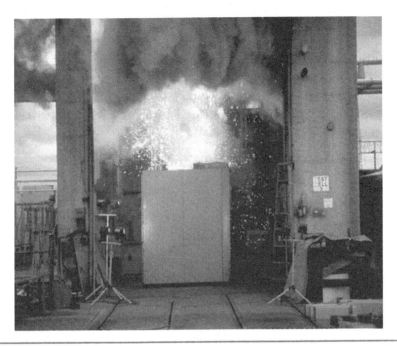

Figure 7.1   An arc blast causes damage from fire, concussion waves, heat, and lique-fied metal.

electrical equipment, which have a melting point of only 1900°F (Figure 7.1).

When copper changes from a solid to a vapor it expands up to 67,000 times its original volume. The expansion causes pressure and sound waves and intense and rapid heating of the surrounding air. The threshold for pressure on your eardrums is 720 lbs/ft^2 and 1728 lbs/ft^2 on your lungs. If the pressure doesn't affect your lungs, inhaling molten metal and vaporized copper will. The next hazard is that equipment components blow apart and expel shrapnel into the arc area at a velocity in excess of 700 miles per hour. So there you are, exposed to temperatures hotter than the sun, breathing in copper vapors, rattled by shrapnel, and being thrown across the room by a shock wave that can rupture your eardrums. We are talking extreme physical devastation here. The severity of these safety hazards prompted action by OSHA to seek protocols to protect workers from the effects of arc flash and arc blasts.

NAPA 70E

There are four separate industry standards that address the prevention of arc flash incidents:

- OSHA 29 Code of Federal Regulations (CFR) Part 1910 Subpart S

- NFPA 70E-2008 National Electrical Code

- NFPA 70E-2009 Standard for Electrical Safety Requirements for Employee Workplaces

- IEEE Standard 1584-2009 Guide for Performing Arc Flash Hazard Calculations

OSHA regulations mandate what electricians have to do in order to have their actions and installations considered safe. I can tell you that you must guard against dangerous electrical conditions, but if I don't tell you how to protect yourself, then how would I ever determine if you were working safely? This was the dilemma facing OSHA, so at the request of OSHA the NFPA committee established NFPA 70E Standard for Electrical Safety Requirements in the Workplace. NFPA 70E identifies a full range of electrical safety issues that OSHA in turn uses as a basis for enforcing its safety mandates. In other words, OSHA tells you what you have to do, NFPA tells you how to do it, and then OSHA measures your compliance with their requirements based on the guidelines established by NFPA 70E.

Some employers think that since the NEC and NFPA 70E are both published by NFPA, they only have to comply with the standards and requirements of the NEC in order to cover all of the bases. Not so. The NEC code consists of standards for electrical design, installation, and inspections. Some provisions in the NEC are not directly related to employee safety. NFPA 70E correlates suitable portions of the NEC with other documents applicable to electrical worker safety. NFPA 70E, not the NEC, provides standards that allow OSHA to enforce safety guidelines for employers and employees in their workplace. Here is an example of how these three publications relate to each other.

OSHA mandates that all services to electrical equipment must be performed in a de-energized state. If it is necessary to perform hot work then the regulations outlined in NFPA 70E, Article 130 should be used as a tool to comply with OSHA mandates Subpart S part 1910.333(a)(1). Employers are also responsible for complying with the 2008 NEC 110.16 labeling requirements which state that *electrical equipment such as* switchboards, panel boards, industrial control panels, and motor control centers have to be field marked to warn qualified persons of potential electric arc flash hazards (Figure 7.2).

This requirement is designed to provide appropriate and consistent applications to field installations that qualify for the warning labels required by this section. The NEC 2008 standard broadened this requirement by including all types of equipment that would qualify for the field-applied arc-flash warning labels. Previously, the requirements of this section were limited to equipment that was actually identified in the rule. By including the words, "equipment such as" the concept is expanded to all equipment types that are likely to require examination, adjustment, servicing, or maintenance while energized. This requirement applies to things like enclosed circuit breakers, some types of transformers, and other equipment that was not specifically included in the previous text. Additionally, the standard puts a limitation on the types of dwelling occupancies in which these labels for

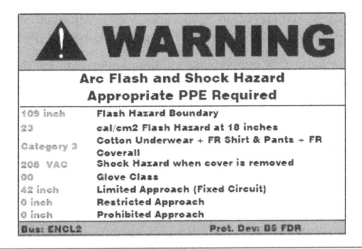

Figure 7.2 Warning labels list approach boundaries and PPE requirements.

equipment are required. For example, multiple occupancy dwelling structures like apartment buildings, where the service equipment and other equipment can be large, require arc-flash warning labels. However, arc-flash warning label requirements do not apply to one- and two-family dwelling units. This specific rule only applies to installations where field-applied arc flash warning labels are required.

The information necessary for these labels is derived from boundary distances calculated in NFPA 70E Article 130. So you can see how important it is for you to understand NFPA 70E safety requirements.

There is no required standard for arc flash label designs.

Article 100 of NFPA 70E lists definitions that are based on installation-related characterizations and NEC terminology. These terms include:

- *Arc rating:* This is the maximum incident energy resistance demonstrated by a material prior to break open.

- *Electrical hazard:* A dangerous condition such as contact or equipment failure that can result in electric shock, arc flash burns, thermal burns, or electrically induced blast.

- *Electrically safe work condition:* A state where the conductor or circuit to be worked on or near has been disconnected from energized parts, locked/tagged in accordance with established standards, tested to ensure the absence of voltage, and grounded if necessary.

- *Flash hazard:* A dangerous condition associated with the release of energy caused by an electrical arc.

- *Flash protection boundary:* An approach limit at a distance from exposed live parts within which a person could receive a second-degree burn if an electrical arc flash were to occur.

- *Incident energy:* The amount of energy impressed on a surface, a certain distance from an energy source, generated during an electrical arc event.

- *Limited approach boundary:* An approach limit at a distance from exposed live parts within which a shock hazard exists.

Article 110.6 addresses specific training requirements for employees who are at risk of encountering electrical hazards. Training must include how to identify potential hazards and determine the degree of risk from these hazards, how each hazard affects the body, and how to avoid exposure to these hazards. Additionally, employees must know how to perform a hazard/risk analysis, chose appropriate personal protective equipment (PPE), ascertain limited, restricted, and prohibited approach boundaries, and how to determine if their actions might result in a release of energy (Figure 7.3).

Determining safe approach distances

How close is too close when you are dealing with electrical hazards? Imagine you have to draw lines on the floor to represent degrees of possible exposure. The line farthest away from live equipment would indicate the limited approach boundary. This is the threshold of the approach distance for unqualified people. Think of it like the bleachers at a football field. Since unqualified people are considered to be less capable or trained in recognizing shock and flash hazards, they need to remain the safest distance possible from the field of hazard posed

Cause and Affect of Trauma Caused by an Electric Arc	
DISTANCE	The amount of damage done to a person is diminished by approximately the square of the distance from the arc. Twice as far away from the arc source equates to one-fourth the damage.
TEMPERATURE	The amount of heat energy received is proportional to the difference between the fourth power of the arc temperature and the body temperature T^4 arc - T^4 body
TIME	The volume of energy received is proportional to the amount of time that the arc is present
ARC LENGTH	The amount of energy transmitted is a result of the arc length. For example, a zero length arc will transmit zero energy.
CROSS-SECTIONAL AREA OF BODY EXPOSED TO THE ARC ANGLE	The greater the area of the body that is exposed, the more energy is received. Energy is proportional to the *sine of the angle of incidence. Energy impinging at 90 degrees is the maximum calculated. *Sine is the ratio of the opposite side of an acute angle in a right triangle

Figure 7.3 The hazards caused by an arc blast are based on factors such as distance from the blast and arc length.

by open, energized conductors. If for some reason an unqualified person needs to cross the limited approach boundary to perform a minor task a qualified person has to ensure they are safe.

Under no circumstances can anyone, even a qualified person, allow an unqualified person to cross a restricted approach boundary.

The restricted approach boundary is the closest distance an unqualified person can be to a shock or flash hazard, like the sidelines of the football field. The only people who are allowed to cross a restricted approach boundary are those who are considered qualified, have an approved approach plan, are wearing appropriate PPE, and who know how to position their bodies in a way that minimizes risk of inadvertent contact with energized conductors. Once you cross this line you are considered to be in the prohibited approach boundary. This is the closest distance to an exposed energized circuit or circuit part that a qualified person can approach (Figure 7.4).

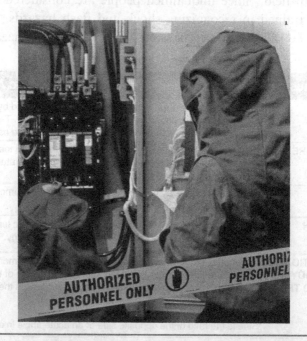

Figure 7.4 Only qualified workers who are wearing appropriate PPE can be within the prohibited boundary. Warning tape or barricades should be used to post the area for authorized personnel only.

If a person crosses this boundary they are looked at as being the same as a person making direct contact with exposed energized parts, and therefore, they have to do the following:

- Have a documented plan that justifies the need to work inside the prohibited approach area, approved by the site manager

- Possess specific training to work on energized conductors or parts

- Have performed a hazard risk analysis, approved by the site manager

- Use PPE appropriate for working on exposed energized parts and rated for the voltage and energy level present (Figure 7.5)

ARC FLASH BOUNDARIES

Arc-flash boundaries need to be established around electrical equipment such as switchboards, panelboards, industrial control panels, motor control centers, and similar equipment if you plan to work on or in the proximity of exposed energized components. Parts are considered exposed if

APPROACH BOUNDARIES TO LIVE PARTS FOR SHOCK PROTECTION				
NOMINAL VOLTAGE RANGE PHASE-TO-PHASE	LIMITED APPROACH BOUNDARY		RESTRICTED APPROACH BOUNDARY	PROHIBITED APPROACH BOUNDARY
	Exposed Movable Conductor	Exposed Fixed Circuit Part	Includes Inadvertent Movement Potential	Qualified personnel only
0 – 50	Not Specified	Not Specified	Not Specified	Not Specified
51 – 300	10 ft	3 ft 6 in	Avoid Contact	Avoid Contact
301 – 750	10 ft	3 ft 6 in	1 ft	1 in
751 – 15 kV	10 ft	5 ft	2 ft 2 in	7 in
15.1 kV – 36 kV	10 ft	6 ft	2 ft 7 in	10 in
36.1 kV – 46 kV	10 ft	8 ft	2 ft 9 in	1 ft 5 in
46.1kV – 72.5 kV	10 ft	8 ft	3 ft 3 in	2 ft 1 in
72.6 kV – 121 kV	10 ft 8 in	8 ft	3 ft 5 in	2 ft 8 in
138 kV – 145 kV	11 ft	10 ft	3 ft 7 in	3 ft 1 in
161 kV – 169 kV	11 ft 8 in	11 ft 8 in	4 ft	3 ft 6 in
230 kV – 242 kV	13 ft	13 ft	5 ft 3 in	4 ft 9 in
345 kV – 362 kV	15 ft 4 in	15 ft 4 in	8 ft 6 in	8 ft
500 kV – 550 kV	19 ft	19 ft	11 ft 3 in	10 ft 9 in
765 kV – 800 kV	23 ft 9 in	23 ft 9 in	14 ft 11 in	14 ft 5 in

Figure 7.5 Approach boundaries are based on the nominal voltage present in energized circuits or parts and whether the exposed hazard is movable or fixed.

they are energized and not enclosed, shielded, covered, or otherwise protected from contact. Work on these parts includes activities such as examinations, adjustment, servicing, maintenance, or troubleshooting.

Equipment energized below 240 V does not require arc-flash boundary calculation unless it is powered by a 112.5 KVA transformer or larger.

The arc-flash boundary is the limit at which a person working on energized parts can be standing at the time of an arc-flash without risking permanent injury unless they are wearing flame-resistant clothing. Permanent injury results from an arc-flash that causes an incident energy of 1.2 calories/centimeter^2 (cal/cm^2) or greater and causes a minimum of second-degree burns. This distance can only be effectively determined by calculating the destructive potential of an arc. First you must determine the magnitude of the arc based on the available short circuit current, then estimate how long the arc will last based on the interrupting time of the fuse or circuit breaker. Finally, you will need to calculate how far away an individual must be to avoid being exposed to an incident energy of 1.2 cal/cm^2. It may sound like a lot of math and factoring in of potentials, but believe me the extra time you take to determine the arc flash boundary is well worth your safety and well-being (Figure 7.6).

Calculating flash protection boundaries for systems over 600 V requires performing a flash hazard analysis coupled with either the NFPA 70E Hazard Risk Category/PPE tables or the Incident Energy Formula. Additionally, Section 4 of IEEE 1584 Guide for Arc Flash Hazard Calculations states that the results of the arc flash hazard analysis are used to identify the flash-protection boundary and the incident energy at assigned working distances throughout any position or level in the overall electrical system. The purpose is to establish safe work distances and the PPE required to protect workers from injury. A flash-hazard analysis is comprised of the following three different electrical system studies:

- A short circuit study

- A protective device time-current coordination study

- The flash-hazard analysis and application of the data

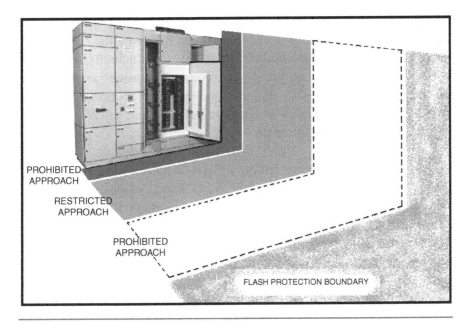

PROHIBITED
APPROACH

RESTRICTED
APPROACH

PROHIBITED
APPROACH

FLASH PROTECTION BOUNDARY

Figure 7.6 Approach boundaries set distance limits for workers based on training levels and the degree of risk.

Arc flash hazard analysis

To perform an arc flash hazard analysis, you need to start by gathering information on the building's power distribution system. This data should include the arrangement of components on a one-line drawing with nameplate specifications of every device on the system and the types and sizes of cables. The local utility company should be contacted so that you can get the minimum and maximum fault currents entering the facility.

Next you will want to perform a short circuit analysis and a coordination study. You will need this information to put into the equations provided in NFPA 70E or the IEEE Standard 1584. These equations will give you the flash protection boundary distances and incident energy potentials you will need to determine your minimum PPE requirements. In many ways an arc fault analysis is actually a study in risk management. You can be very conservative in your analysis and the results will almost always indicate the need for category 4 PPE. On the other hand, you can perform the analysis and make adjustments to reduce the arc fault conditions resulting in reduced PPE requirements. However, use caution when adjusting your calculations. Reducing the bolted fault current can reduce the arc fault current, but it can actually result in a worse situation. For example, if you reduce the current applied to a motor from 4000 to 1800 A, the arc fault energy is increased from 0.6 to 78.8 cal/cm^2. This is the exact opposite outcome that you might expect to achieve before doing the math.

Keep in mind that you are risking OSHA violations and fines if you choose nominal compliance. On the other hand, you can actually be increasing the risk of injury if you force workers to unnecessarily wear cumbersome PPE. This can also result in little or no high voltage maintenance being performed, which will eventually compromise safety and proper equipment operation. It might prove beneficial to get a registered professional engineering firm to perform arc flash hazard calculations on your behalf and have them recommend appropriate actions and the lowest appropriate category of PPE.

SHORT-CIRCUIT STUDY

A short circuit is any current that is not confined to its normal, intended path. The term is derived from the fact that these currents bypass, or find a "short" path, around the normal load. Short circuits are usually caused by accidental contact or worn or damaged insulation and are more serious than overloads because damage occurs almost instantly. Typical examples of events that cause a short circuit are someone touching or dropping tools across energized conductors, inadvertently touching a hot load, or accidental connection between energized conductors and ground.

Circuit breakers can take up to 12 times longer to open than current limiting fuses under short circuit conditions.

A short-circuit study estimates short-circuit potential and is based on a review of one-line drawings which will need to be field-verified. If these drawings don't exist, they will have to be created. The maximum available fault current is calculated at each significant point in the system. Each interrupting protective device is analyzed to determine whether it is appropriately designed and sized to interrupt the circuit in the event of a bolted type of short circuit. Next, all associated equipment is reviewed to ensure that the bus bars are adequately braced to handle the available fault current. Finally, the bolted fault currents are converted into arc fault currents for additional analysis.

It's really important to obtain the minimum available short circuit current as well as the maximum short circuit current from the electric utility. Voltage fluctuations in a site's power supply have to be taken into consideration when you are developing the short circuit calculations. Arc fault calculations need to be evaluated at more than just the worst-case conditions (Figure 7.7).

COORDINATION STUDY

A coordination study is the examination of the electrical system and available documentation with the goal of ensuring that overcurrent protection devices are properly designed and coordinated. An overload is defined as an excessive or overcurrent power draw that is confined to the normal current path. Most conductors are capable of carrying a moderate overload for a short time without damage and overcurrent protection devices can be used that will carry these currents. However,

ARC FLASH EQUATIONS

ENERGY (E)   = POWER (P) x TIME (t)

POWER (P)   = VOLTS (V) x AMPS (I)

CALORIES (E) = VOLTS (V) x AMPS (I) x TIME (T)

1 Calorie   = 4.1868 watt-seconds

1 Joule   = 1 watt-second

Figure 7.7 Equations used in calculating arc flash hazards.

excessive loads, stalled motors, or overloaded machine tools can call for too much current and overload a circuit. If an overload occurs and exceeds the protection devices or lasts for too long, excessive heat will be generated that will ultimately cause insulation failure. This action can lead to a fire or a short circuit.

The first step in conducting a coordination study is to rate all overcurrent protective devices, and select and adjust them so that only the fault current carrying device nearest a potential fault opens to isolate a faulted circuit from the system. These adjustments are made so that pickup currents and operating times are as short as possible while remaining sufficient enough to override system transient overloads such as inrush currents experienced when energizing transformers or starting motors. In this way, the rest of the system will remain in operation, providing maximum service continuity. The study consists of time-current coordination curves that illustrate coordination among the devices that are shown on the one-line diagram (Figure 7.8).

Let's look at an example of establishing a flash boundary using the Hazard Risk Category/PPE table from NFPA 70E. Assume we have an overcurrent protective device with a clearing time of six cycles or less and an available fault current of 50 kA, or any combination where the product of the clearing time and the available fault current does not exceed 300 kA cycles or 5000 A s. This equates to a flash boundary of 4 feet based on wearing the PPE listed in the table provided in NFPA 70E Article 130.7.

To use the incident energy formula for clearing times and bolted fault currents greater than 300 kA cycles you will need the bolted fault current and the transformer capacity rating. The formula looks like this:

$$D_c = [2.65 \times MVA_{bf} \times t]^{1/2}$$

OR

$$D_c = [53 \times MVA \times t]^{1/2}$$

D_c = The distance in feet from an arc source in which a second degree burn would occur.

MVA_{bf} = The bolted fault capacity available at the contact point, measured in mega-volt-amps. This capacity is expressed in millions of volt-amps.

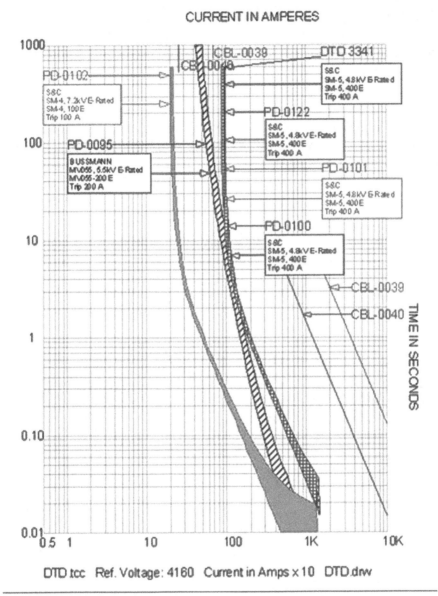

Figure 7.8   An example of a coordination curve.

MVA = The bolted fault capacity available at the possible point of contact. Measured in mega-volt-amps, for transformers with MVA ratings below 0.75 MVA, multiply the MVA rating by 1.25.

The critical variable in these formulas is time. When electrical energy is released it escalates rapidly. For this reason, an arc flash boundary is dependent on the characteristics of an overcurrent protection device (Figure 7.9).

These overcurrent devices should be selected so they limit the arc time duration and current magnitude. When the potential fault current is within the current-limiting range of current-limiting fuses, the arc flash hazard potential is reduced. The thermal energy potential that an arcing flash would release also needs to be determined in order to choose the appropriate PPE.

Older existing breakers with slow reaction times that trip at too high a current can be replaced with more modern breakers. The new breakers can be adjusted to trip earlier than before. This can limit the flash hazard and result in many category 4 PPE requirements being decreased to category 1 or 2.

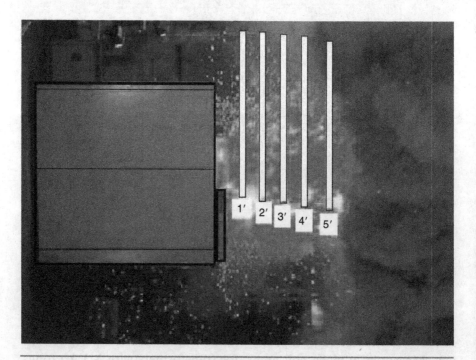

Figure 7.9 Electrical arc flash extends over a significant distance in a short time.

NFPA 70E Article 130.3 requires a flash hazard analysis, and provides the formulas necessary for determining hazard risk categories and the corresponding required PPE in NFPA 70E Table 130.(C)(9)(a) (Figure 7.10).

Arc-Flash Hazard Calculations **Example using Littlefuse Class L 2500 Amp Fuses**	
Step 1:	Review one line drawing and determine the available short circuit current and other details about the location of the equipment.
Step 2:	Our one line drawing states that the 2000kVA transformer has a 4160V primary and 480V secondary with 5.5% impedance.
Step 3:	We need to determine the MVAbf of the transformer. Since 2000kVA is 2 MVA, the MVAbf = MVA 100 /%Z or 2 × 100 / 5.5 = 36.4 MVA.
Step 4:	Calculate the clearing time of the 2500 Amp Class L fuse at the fault current. The maximum three phase bolted fault current at the transformer secondary is determined by the formula: Isc = (MVA × 106 × 100) / 3 × 480 × 5.5 = 43,738 Amps = 43.7 kA. The time current curve for the Littelf use 2500 Amp Class L fuse indicates the clearing time at 43,738 Amps is 0.01 second = ta
Step 5:	Determine the Flash Protection Boundary (FPB) using the formula in NFPA 70E Article 130.3(A). In Step 3, we determined that MVAbf is 36.4 and ta = 0.01 second, so we use these values in the equation: Dc = [2.65 × MVAbf × t]½ Therefore, Dc = [2.65 × 36.4 × 0.01]½ = 0.98 ft. (~12 inches)
Step 6:	Calculate the Incident Energy at **18 inches** working distance using the NFPA 70E formula for "Arc-in-a-box" listed in Annex D 6.2(a)] as follows: DB = 18 (inches) ta = 0.01 and F (from Step 4) = 43.7 Therefore, EMB = 1038.7 DB −1.4738 × ta[0.0093F 2−0.3453F+5.9675] EMB = 1038.7 × (18)−1.4738 × (.01) × [0.0093(43.7)2 − 0.3453(43.7)+5.9675] **EMB = 1.27 cal/cm²**
Step 7:	Determine the Hazard Risk Category with Littelfuse 2500 Amp Class L fuse. Since the Incident Energy is 1.27 cal/cm² at 18 inches, NFPA 70E Table 130.7(C)(11) defines the minimum Arc Rating of PPE up to 4 cal/cm² as **Hazard Risk Category 1.**

Figure 7.10 Hazard risk categories are determined based on the types of overcurrent protection, current, and incident energy.

Arc-Flash Hazard Calculations
Example using 2500 Amp Low Voltage Power Circuit Breaker

Step 1:	Determine the clearing time of the circuit breaker at the fault level. Isc = 43,738 Amps, and the time current curve for the Circuit Breaker shows **t** (the clearing time) is 5 cycles = 0.083 second.
Step 2:	Determine the Flash Protection Boundary using NFPA 70E Article 130.3(A) formula: The MVAbf of our transformer is 36.4 and t = 0.083 second Dc = [2.65 × MVAbf × t]½ Therefore, Dc = [2.65 × 36.4 × .083]½ = 2.83 ft. (34 inches)
Step 3:	Calculate the Incident Energy at **18 inches** working distance with the circuit breaker using the NFPA 70E formula for "Arc-in-a-box" listed in Annex D 6.2(a)] We established that DB =18 (inches) and ta= 0.083 and F= 43.7 (kA) Therefore:EMB = 1038.7 DB −1.4738 ta[0.0093F2−0.3453F+5.9675] EMB = 1038.7 × (18)−1.4738 × (0.083) × [0.0093(43.7)2− 0.3453(43.7) + 5.9675] **EMB = 10.54 cal/cm²**
Step 4:	Determine the Hazard Risk Category. Since the Incident Energy is at 18 inches and NFPA Table 130.7(C)(11) defines the minimum Arc Rating of PPE up to.
Step 5:	Determine the Hazard Risk Category using 2500 Amp circuit breaker. Since the Incident Energy is 10.54 cal/cm² at 18 inches, NFPA 70E Table 130.7(C)(11) defines the minimum Arc Rating of PPE up to 25 cal/cm² as **Hazard Risk Category 3.**

Figure 7.10—Cont'd

Personal protective equipment

When it comes to preventing injury from arc incidents, your PPE needs to consist of more than a hardhat and a pair of work boots. OSHA Part 1910.335(a) requires that employees working in areas where there are potential electrical hazards have and use electrical protective equipment that is appropriate for specific parts of the body to be protected and for the work to be performed. The purpose of PPE is to protect individuals exposed to health and safety hazards from the risk of injury by creating a barrier against various hazards.

A wide range of protective gear exists, including:

- Nonconductive flame-resistant head, face, and chin protection, including hardhats, full face shields, and switching hoods

- Eye protection such as face shields, safety glasses, and goggles

- Hand and arm protection such as insulating gloves and sleeves with leather coverings

- Foot and leg protection using insulated leg and footwear

- Full body equipment including flash resistant shirts, pants, jackets, and coveralls

- Insulating blankets or mats (Figure 7.11)

With such a variety of protection available, exactly what equipment is considered "appropriate" is defined in NFPA 70E. This is determined by the task to be performed and the risks present in the type of work you will be doing. In order to figure out the risks you may be exposed to, you needed to analyze the potential hazards. Armed with the results of your flash hazard analysis, you are ready to match your risk to the PPE that NFPA 70E has deemed suitable for the work you need to perform.

Before we look at how to determine the level of PPE required for various types of work, let's take a minute to get acclimated with a few terms that pertain to PPE.

- *Arc thermal performance exposure value (ATPV):* The incident energy level, measured in cal/cm^2, which can cause the onset of a second-degree burn as defined in ASTM F 1959 Standard Test Method for Determining the Arc Thermal Performance Value of Materials for Clothing. PPE is rated and labeled with a calorie rating, such as 11 cal/cm^2.

- *Calories per centimeter squared:* This is a number that indicates the amount of energy that can be delivered to a given point at a particular distance from an explosion. Once this value is

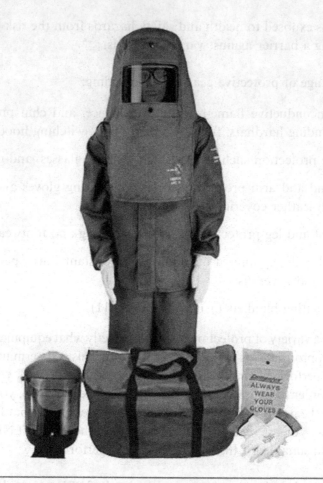

Figure 7.11 A protective arc suit and flash helmet.

known, the ATPV rating required for work analyzed at that distance from the potential flash hazard is determined. Cal/cm^2 are the units of incident energy that the PPE can withstand.

■ *Energy break open threshold (EBT):* This is the term used to describe the physical strength of fabric as it applies to the material's ability to withstand thermal energy. The incident energy level that doesn't cause flame resistant (FR) fabric to fail, or break open, and does not exceed second-degree burn criteria, as defined in ASTM F 1959. It is also extremely important to avoid contamination of PPE material. Contact with grease, solvents, and flammable liquids may destroy the protection.

■ *Fabric weight:* This is usually represented in one of two ways: ounces per square yard or grams per square meter. Both of these values essentially refer to the thickness of the fabric. The more ounces per square yard, the more material exists in the same square yard of fabric.

■ *Flame resistant:* The property of a material whereby combustion is prevented, terminated, or inhibited following the application of a flaming or non-flaming source of ignition, with or without subsequent removal of the ignition source (Figure 7.12).

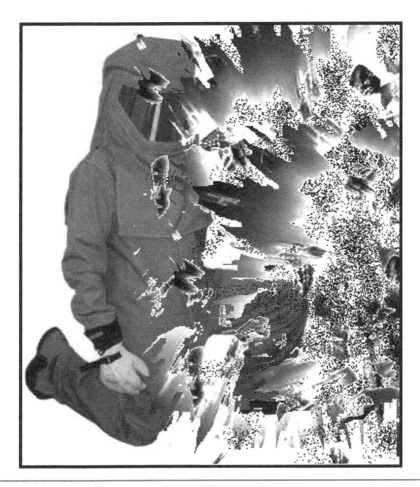

Figure 7.12 The ATPV rating and flame resistance of PPE. Arc suits do not eliminate damage from shock waves or shrapnel.

- *Heat attenuation factor (HAF):* This is the amount of heat blocked by a fabric. Just because a fabric is 10% FR does not mean it will block all of the heat to which it could be exposed. An HAF of 85% means that the material will block 85% of the heat the fabric encounters. This is based on exposure to a short burst of heat, typically less than 1 s. In the event of prolonged heat exposure, the HAF would be much lower.

- *V-rated:* Voltage rating. Tools and gloves are rated and tested for the line-to-line voltage at the area where the work is to be performed.

OSHA 1910.137 specifies that protective gear must be maintained and periodically inspected to ensure that it remains in a safe and reliable condition. NFPA 70E Articles 130.7(B), 130.7(C)(8), and 130.7(F) also require that PPE must be inspected before and after each use, and be repaired, cleaned, or laundered according to the manufacturer's instructions prior to use.

The minimum level of a required PPE would be an untreated natural fiber long-sleeve shirt and long pants with safety glasses with side shields. This would be a hazard risk category of 0, while a rating of 4 is the most hazardous scenario. Figure 7.13 is a quick reference for PPE based on risk categories, by incident energy.

Risk/Hazard Category	Incident Energy Cal/cm^2	PPE Required - Clothing
0	Up to 2	Untreated Cotton (non-melting clothing)
1	>2 up to 4	Flame retardant (FR) shirt and FR pants
2	4-8	Cotton underwear + FR shirt and FR pants
3	8 to 25	Cotton underwear + FR shirt, FR pants and FR coveralls
4	25 to 40	Cotton underwear + FR shirt, FR pants and double layer switching coat and pants

Figure 7.13 Risk categories based on incident determine the type of protective clothing required.

Additional PPE that can be required includes safety boots, face shields, and leather over voltage-rated gloves. NFPA 70E Table 3-3.9.2 groups these articles of protective clothing and equipment by category rating. For example, a hardhat and side shield safety glasses or goggles are required for every category of work from 1 to 4. However, a flame-resistant hardhat liner must be added for category 3 or 4 tasks. On the other hand, a two-layer flash suit jacket and pants are only needed for category 4 work. It is important to know the basic PPE that makes up each category. Figure 7.15 provides a quick reference chart (Figure 7.14).

WHAT NOT TO WEAR

A second-degree burn can occur with only 1.2 cal/cm^2 of incident energy. A number of clothing materials are considered highly flammable or dangerous because the material can actually melt when exposed to high temperatures. Many synthetic materials fall into this category, including acetate, nylon, polyester, and rayon or blends that include these materials. Consider the fact that incident energy is a radiant energy that will pass through even FR material and can ignite or heat underclothing to the point where a burn results. A little humor can be used when addressing this delicate subject. Our company's motto was, when you have to do hot work wear your tightie whities or your granny

TYPE OF CLOTHING and EQUIPMENT	PPE CATEGORY			
	1	2	3	4
Hardhat	X	X	X	X
Eye protection (safety glasses + side shields or safety goggles)	X	X		
Leather gloves	As Needed	X		
Face protection (double-layer switching hood)		2* tasks	X	X
Hearing protection (ear canal inserts)		2* tasks	X	X
Voltage-rated gloves with leather protectors			X	X
Flash suit jacket (2-layer)				X
Flash suit pants (2-layer)				X

Figure 7.14 Types of PPE by category.

Hazard/Risk Category Classification (within flash protection boundary)

TASK:	PPE Category	V-R Gloves	V-R Tools
OPENING DOORS AND COVERS			
Open hinged covers (to expose bare, energized parts)			
240 volts or less	0	N	N
600-volt-class motor control centers	1	N	N
600-volt-class lighting or small power transformers	1	N	N
600-volt-class switchgear (with power circuit breakers or fused switches)	2	N	N
NEMA E2 (fused contactor) motor starters, 2.3 kV through 7.2 kV	3	N	N
1 kV and over (metal clad switchgear)	3	N	N
1 kV and higher, (metal clad load interrupter switches, fused or unfused)	3	N	N
Remove bolted covers (expose bare, energized parts)			
240 volts or less	1	N	N
600-volt-class motor control centers or transformers	2*	N	N
600-volt-class lighting or small power transformers	2*	N	N
600-volt-class switchgear (with power circuit breakers or fused switches)	3	N	N
NEMA E2 (fused contactor) motor starters, 2.3 kV through 7.2 kV	4	N	N
1 kV and higher (metal clad switchgear)	4	N	N
1 kV and higher, (metal clad load interrupter switches, fused or unfused)	4	N	N
Open transformer compartments (metal clad switchgear 1 kV and higher)	4	N	N

Figure 7.15 Hazard/Risk Category Classification (within flash protection boundary).

panties. It may sound too personal to discuss, but if you wear silky boxers or panties you could end up wearing them adhered to your skin for the rest of your life.

Table method of what to wear

Before determining the appropriate PPE for the work to be performed, you must identify the equipment that will be worked on. Then you need to review the up-to-date one line drawing for information about the available short circuit current and other details about the location of the equipment.

TASK:	PPE Category	V-R Gloves	V-R Tools
INSTALLING, REMOVING, OPERATING : **Circuit Breakers (CBs), Fused Switches, Motor Starters or Fused Contactors**			
Installing or removing circuit breakers or fused switches, 240 volts or less	1	Y	Y
Insert or remove (rack) CBs from cubicles, doors closed			
600-volt switchgear (with power circuit breakers or fused switches)	2	N	N
NEMA E2 (fused contactor) motor starters, 2.3 kV through 7.2 kV	2	N	N
1 kV and higher (metal clad switchgear)	2	N	N
Insert or remove (rack) CBs or starters from cubicles, doors open			
600-volt-class switchgear (with power circuit breakers or fused switches)	3	N	N
NEMA E2 (fused contactor) Motor Starters, 2.3 kV through 7.2 kV	3	N	N
1 kV and higher (metal clad switchgear)	4	N	N
Operate circuit breaker (CB), fused switch, motor			
240 volts or less	0	N	N
Over 240 but less than 600 volt panelboards	1	N	N
600 volt class motor control centers	1	N	N
600 volt class switchgear (with power circuit breakers or fused switches)	1	N	N
NEMA E2 (fused contactor) motor starters, 2.3 kV through 7.2 kV	2*	N	N
1 kV and higher (metal clad switchgear)	4	N	N
2* = A double-layer switching hood and hearing protection are required, in addition to the other hazard/risk category 2 requirements of table 3-3.9.2 of Part II of NFPA 70E.			

Figure 7.15—Cont'd

Next, you can try to use the table method provided by NFPA 70E Table 130.7(C)(9)(a) to match the type of work you will be performing. If the task you need to complete is not listed in the table, you have no option but to complete a flash hazard analysis to determine PPE. If the type of work is listed, use the table to identify the hazard risk category associated with the task and determine if voltage rated gloves or tools are required (Figure 7.15).

Be sure to check the conditions listed in the footnotes for NFPA 70E Table 30.7(C)(9)(a) to see if they are applicable to the work you will

TASK:	PPE Category	V-R Gloves	V-R Tools
WORK ON ENERGIZED PARTS			
Work on energized parts, voltage testing, applying safety grounds			
240 volts or less	1	Y	Y
Over 240 but less than 600 volt panelboards	2*	Y	Y
600-volt-class motor control centers	2*	Y	Y
600-volt-class switchgear (with power circuit breakers or fused switches)	2*	Y	Y
600-volt-class lighting or small power transformers	2*	Y	Y
600-volt-class revenue meters	2*	Y	Y
NEMA E2 (fused contactor) motor starters, 2.3 kV through 7.2 kV	3	Y	Y
1 kV and higher (metal clad switchgear)	4	Y	Y
1 kV and higher metal clad load interrupter switches, fused or unfused	4	Y	Y
Work on control circuits with exposed energized parts, 120 volts or below			
600-volt-class motor control centers	0	Y	Y
600-volt-class switchgear (with power circuit breakers or fused switches	0	Y	Y
NEMA E2 (fused contactor) motor starters, 2.3 kV through 7.2 kV	0	Y	Y
1 kV and higher (metal clad switchgear)	2	Y	Y
Work on control circuits with exposed energized parts, over 120 volts			
600-volt-class motor control centers	2*	Y	Y
600-volt-class switchgear (with power circuit breakers or fused switches)	2*	Y	Y
NEMA E2 (fused contactor) motor starters, 2.3 kV through 7.2 kV	3	Y	Y
1 kV and higher (metal clad switchgear)	4	Y	Y
2* = A double-layer switching hood and hearing protection are required, in addition to the other hazard/risk category 2 requirements of table 3-3.9.2 of Part II of NFPA 70E.			
Applying safety grounds after voltage testing does not require voltage-rated tools. Voltage-rated gloves or tools are rated and tested for the maximum line-to-line voltage on which work will be done. The hazard/risk category may be reduced by one number for low-voltage equipment listed here where the short-circuit current available is less than 15 kA (less than 25 kA for 600-volt-class switchgear).			

Figure 7.15—Cont'd Low-voltage tasks (600 V and below). This sample chart applies when there is an available short-circuit capacity of 25 kA or less, and when the fault clearing time is 0.03 s (two cycles) or less. For 600-volt-class motor control centers, a short-circuit current capacity of 65 kA or less and fault-clearing time of 0.33 s (20 cycles) is permitted. For 600-volt-class switchgear, a short-circuit current capacity of 65 kA or less and fault-clearing time of 1 s (60 cycles) is used.

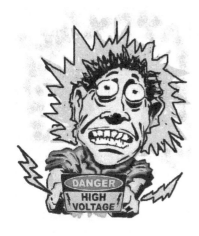

ARC BLAST
CHECK LIST

✓ **De-energize electrical equipment** before work is performed, unless de-energizing would create a hazard.

✓ **Establish an electrical safety program with clearly defined responsibilities,** such as lock out/tag out procedures, names of qualified workers, and any internal safety policies.

✓ **Conduct an electrical system Hazard Analysis** to determine arc flash potential hazards. An arc flash analysis will determine the incident energy potential of each piece of electrical distribution equipment involved in a facility.

✓ **Determine the Hazard/Risk Category of PPE** that is required for workers while performing any work when energized parts are exposed, as defined by the incident energy potential established during the Hazard Analysis.

✓ **Determine "Qualified" workers** who have the skills and knowledge related to the electrical equipment and systems, and have received safety training on the hazards involved.

✓ **Ensure the proper tools and personal protective clothing are available** including fire-resistant shirts, pants or coveralls, a multilayer flash suit, insulated voltage rated hand tools, and insulated voltage measuring devices that are properly rated or the voltage to be tested.

✓ **Apply warning labels to all equipment** to any switchboards, panel boards, control panels, meter socket enclosures and motor control centers.

Figure 7.00   An Arc Blast check list can be instrumental in protecting against blast injuries.

be doing. Then you can use NFPA 70E Tables 130.7(C)(10-11) and the corresponding notes in Table 130.7(C)(9)(a) to properly determine the required PPE for the task at hand.

You must determine the flash protection boundary, even though it is not listed in Table NFPA 70E. For systems 600 V and below, NFPA 70E defines the FPB as 4 feet.

Most people who work around energized equipment have heard stories about arc flashes, but few have seen one in person. Unfortunately, this can lead to an attitude of "it will never happen to me." Remember this—an arc flash or blast incident is a very grim situation, and if you do not utilize the proper precautions it will result in serious, often permanent or terminal, injuries. Working on energized equipment can be done safely if you are properly prepared for arc flash hazards and are aware of how to reduce the risks (Figure 7.00).

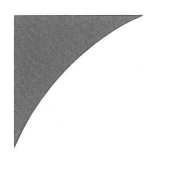

Specific Requirements of the NESC

Published by the IEEE, the National Electrical Safety Code (NESC®) establishes rules to safeguard workers during the installation, operation, or maintenance of electric supply and communication lines and associated equipment. The purpose of the NESC is to provide practical safeguard methods for both utility workers and the public during the installation, operation, and maintenance of electric supply and **171** communication lines and equipment. The major risk hazard in this type of work is the high voltage involved in supplying power from stations and substations to property locations. Some of the requirements for electrical supply structures, equipment, and locations share basic similarities to standards for residential, commercial, and industrial systems covered in the NEC.

High voltage power is intrinsically dangerous and results in injuries that are often catastrophic and frequently fatal. It is not just utility workers who are at risk from high voltage power. Anyone working around power lines needs to be mindful not to inadvertently come in contact with the energized circuits. This includes people working on roofs, scaffolding, and bucket trucks and dump trucks. Even though the NESC provides specific clearance requirements for line installations and clearances, a number of circumstances can occur on construction sites that create hazards. For example, at one New England construction site several winter storms had resulted in a large pile of snow next to a commercial construction site. Snowplows drove over the snow repeatedly and compacted the snow several feet thick. A dump truck arrived at the site to deliver a load of crushed stone and, because the top of the snow level was now much higher than the original level of the ground, the dump truck bed contacted overhead power lines when it was raised up. In this case, the power lines had been installed properly; however, the dump truck operator did not take the time to notice that there were overhead lines before he engaged the dump body. This is a perfect example of why anyone working near power lines must be mindful of clearances and currents.

Electric supply installations

High voltage hazards originate at the point of power generation, which is often the electric supply station. Supply stations are required to be enclosed or fenced to restrict access by unqualified workers. Mechanical parts that are located inside a station must also be safeguarded or isolated. NESC 123 requires protective grounding of all non-current carrying metal parts. If a conductor, bus section, or equipment is disconnected for maintenance purposes, it must also be grounded with either permanent grounding switches or portable grounding jumpers (Figure 8.1).

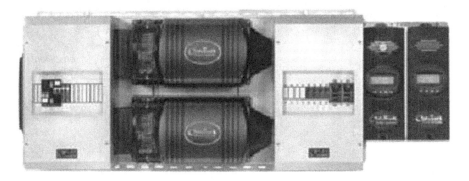

Figure 8.1 Grounded bus bars can be used in a power station to protect non-current carrying metal parts.

NESC Table 124-1 is used to determine the required clearances to energized parts in an electric supply station. Additionally, Rule 124A3 specifies an 8 foot 6 inch clearance requirement to parts with an indeterminate potential. This is the space between the top and bottom of a bushing that has an unknown voltage. The required clearance to live parts in the station is determined based on vertical and/or horizontal clearances. If substation equipment is located on a concrete pad that is large enough to stand on, then the clearance measurement is taken from the top of the concrete pad. Otherwise, the measurement is made from the substation surface.

The NESC does not specify bus-to-bus clearance, conductor to bus clearance, or conductor-to-conductor clearance. Instead, "accepted good practices" are to be used. ANSI C37.32 and NEMA SG6 are used to define accepted good practice.

CURRENT AND VOLTAGE TRANSFORMERS

Electric supply stations generate power. Transformers transfer electric energy from one alternating-current circuit to one or more other circuits, either increasing (stepping up) or reducing (stepping down) the voltage. A current transformer (CT) is used for the measurement of electric currents (Figure 8.2).

CTs are commonly used in metering and protective relays in the electrical power industry. A voltage transformer (VT), sometimes known as a

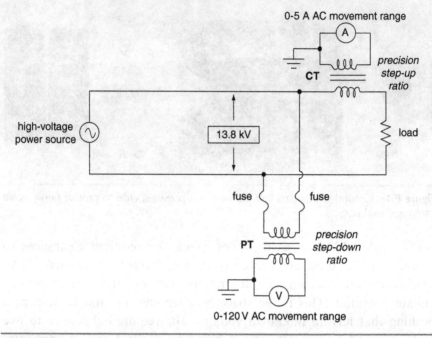

Figure 8.2   A schematic of a typical current transformer.

potential transformer (PT), converts supply voltage to a voltage level suitable for a meter. In this type of transformer, the secondary voltage is substantially proportional to the primary voltage and differs in phase from it by an angle that is approximately zero for an appropriate direction of the connections (Figure 8.3).

The secondary circuits of a CT have to be protected, typically by metal conduit, and secondaries of both CTs and VTs must be effectively grounded. This safety protocol protects against dangerously high voltages and arcing that could occur in open or damaged secondary circuits. Additionally, electric supply station power transformers require a means of automatically disconnecting short-circuit protection.

CONDUCTORS

Conductors in an electrical supply station have to be suitable for the location, use, and voltage, and must be sized to provide adequate ampacity. Compliance is based on the ampacity table in the NEC,

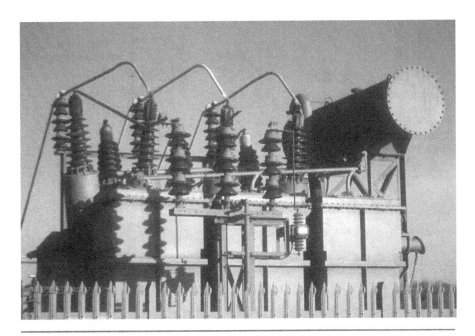

Figure 8.3   A voltage transformer is used to convert high voltage supply current to a lower voltage.

which is also used to determine fuse and circuit breaker sizes. For example, a 120-volt, 20-amp, single-pole, thermal-magnetic circuit breaker used to protect a #12 American wire gauge (AWG) copper, 600-volt conductor serves as both overload protection by means of the circuit breaker thermal element and as short-circuit protection via the breaker's magnetic element.

An electrical protection device may protect the conductor as well as a piece of equipment. For example, the high-side fuse of a substation transformer can also serve as short-circuit protection for the substation bus bars and transformer.

SURGE ARRESTERS

Surge arresters are used to protect equipment in electric utility systems from overvoltage due to switching surges. In electric supply stations, surge arrestors are used to limit damage to vital equipment such as

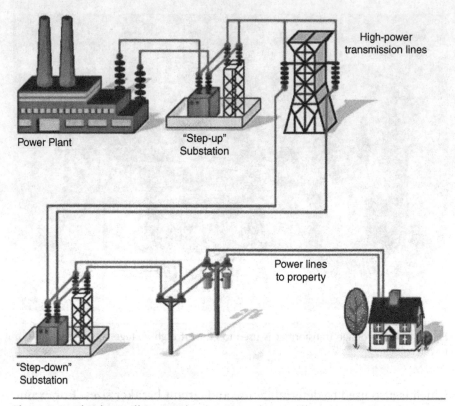

Figure 8.4 This figure illustrates the transition of power from the source at the power supply station to residential use.

power transformers. Surge arrestors should be installed as close as possible to the equipment they protect. Because these arrestors can discharge hot gases and produce electrical arcs, they need to be located away from combustible or energized parts (Figure 8.4).

Communication lines

Communication lines can be affected by voltages induced by power supply lines. However, clearance requirements between power and communication lines are designed for safety, not to eliminate induced voltage. Multiple communication lines on the same structure that are exposed to power contacts, induction, or lightning have to be bonded together, while single communication messengers have to be effectively grounded. If a guy insulator separates a guy, it must be placed on the guy no less than 8 inches above the ground level. Insulators also have to be installed on a guy in a manner that will not permit voltage transfer to the power facility if the guy comes in contact with an energized part or conductor. You also need to install insulators so that if the guy sags down the insulator will not become ineffective.

The communication lines themselves must also be protected by insulation if the conductors exceed 300 V to ground or carry a steady-state induced voltage of a hazardous level. Additional protection should be provided by surge arrestors in conjunction with fusible elements as necessary when severe conditions, such as large supply station current, exist.

Communication circuits that are located in the same space on a pole as the power supply must be installed and maintained by a qualified person per NESC Sections 42 and 44.

Communication lines belonging to different utilities require a clearance of 4 inches between the cables. This keeps communication circuits owned by one company from sagging onto or below communication circuits owned by another utility company. You are not required to take the temperature of loading conditions and variations into consideration when you determine the required 4 inches. However, if the two independent utility companies agree, they can waive the 4-inch clearance requirement. The clearance standard for separate communication lines is covered under Rule 235H2.

Overhead power lines

In order to be considered current carrying, conductors must be connected to a voltage source. A conductor that is used as a common neutral for primary and secondary circuits must be effectively grounded. Line or service conductors that are not neutrals and which are intentionally grounded must meet the requirements of NESC Section 09. If a surge arrestor depends on a ground connection, it must be grounded. An example of a non-dependent surge arrestor would be one across the phase bushings of a voltage regulator. Non-current carrying parts are items such as guy wires. Guys have to be effectively grounded or insulated; however, you cannot use only the guy anchor as a grounding method. Other non-current carrying parts that need to be effectively grounded include metal parts, lampposts, conduits and raceways, cable sheaths, metal switch handles, and operating rods.

You do not want just anyone climbing up a power pole or lattice tower. For this reason, there needs to be 8 feet between pole steps and standoff brackets. This creates a "not readily climbable" support structure and meets the requirements of NESC Section 02.

When you layout power lines for support structures, caution should be used to avoid conflict between various types of lines, such as supply phase lines and communications lines. An ideal configuration that achieves sufficient separation of lines would be as follows:

- Starting at the top of the pole, install power supply phase and neutral lines

- Moving down the pole, install communications lines such as cable TV and telephone (Figure 8.5)

The phase and neutral power lines that run on the same structure are considered "collinear construction." The term "joint use construction" would apply to two or more different kinds of utilities that use the same structure, such as the power lines combined with the communication lines. The basic rule of thumb is to separate lines based on the type of circuit, total number and weight of conductors, the number of branches (taps) and service drops, and any encroaching obstacles such as trees or right of ways.

POWER LINE SPANS

Probably the most frequently referenced part of the NESC is Rule 232 in Section 23, which refers to vertical clearance requirements for above ground wires, cables, conductors, and equipment. Two of the most important clearance safety considerations are sag and tension of conductors. Sag results from environmental elements such as wind, ice, as well as conductor temperature, and is influenced by support structure spans. Sag values are commonly calculated at the center of a span.

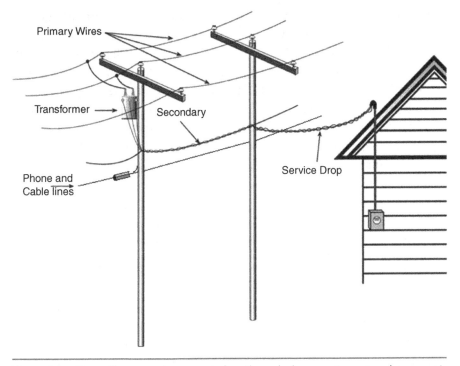

Figure 8.5 Power lines must be separated on the pole from equipment and communication lines.

A "ruling span" is the span that governs, or rules, the actions of all of the spans between two conductor deadends. Span lengths are critical in correctly calculating tension and sag potentials.

The first step in determining line clearances is to calculate the ruling span by using a formula based on span lengths between the conductor deadends. Each span is assigned a consecutive number where S1, S2, S3... are the span lengths between deadends as illustrated in the following formula:

$$\text{RULING SPAN} = \sqrt{\frac{S_1^3 + S_2^3 + S_3^3}{S_1 + S_2 + S_3}}$$

The NESC contains a sag and tension chart based on a span length that is equal to the ruling span, but to estimate the sag for spans that are longer or shorter than the ruling span, use this formula:

$$\text{Sag in feet} = \left(\frac{\text{Span length}}{\text{Ruling span length}}\right)^2 \times \text{Ruling span sag in feet}$$

Conductor temperatures are based on the amount of electrical current carried by the conductor and environmental factors such as the ambient air temperature, cooling effects of wind, and radiant heating effects of the sun. The maximum sag for a conductor usually occurs at 32°F with ice, 120°F final, or greater than 120°F. The minimum tension occurs at the maximum sag due to the high temperatures at the final tension point. Increasing tension will decrease sag. Characteristics of the conductor that affect sag and tension calculations include the AWG rating, cross-sectional area (Area), diameter (Dia), weight (Wt), and rated tensile strength (RTS).

> The phase and neutral conductor of the same circuit may operate at different temperatures because they can carry different levels of electrical current. For this reason, you need to consider them separately from the power conductor.

Ice and wind conditions are divided into three geographical location zones. Zone 1 includes the north central and northeast areas of the United States and Alaska. Zone 2 consists of the northwestern, mid-central, and mid-eastern portions of the United States. Zone 3 is comprised of the southwestern, south central, and southeastern areas of the U.S. These loads are used to determine the physical loading limits for conductors; however, sag is checked at the ice condition only provided in NESC Table 230-1. The minimum permissible sag clearance for phase conductors is 18 feet 5 inches from any point, not just the mid-span. For the neutral conductor, the minimum sag is 15 feet 5 inches, and 16 feet for any secondary duplex, triplex, or quadruplex lines. Communication line sag cannot be less than 15 feet 5 inches to any roads, streets, or other travel areas that could support truck traffic (Figure 8.6).

SUPPLY EMPLOYEE SAFETY

Sections 42 and 44 relate to worker safety guidelines and requirements. Personal protection precautions are provided regarding protective devices, equipment, and guidelines. For example, the section on emergency methods indicates that all power line workers should be familiar with first aid, rescue techniques, and fire extinguishing methods.

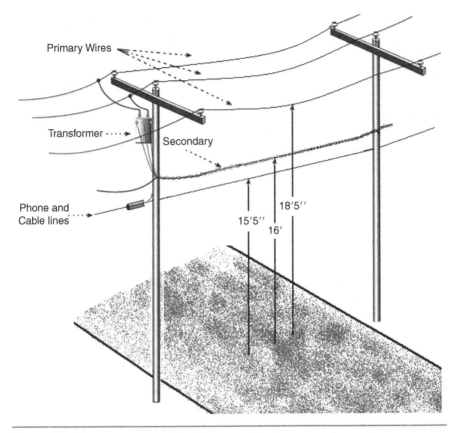

Figure 8.6 Clearances are required to account for line sag and separation.

Section 42 also explains your responsibility to safeguard yourself and others. You are required to report any line or equipment defects, such as low clearances and broken insulators, observed while working on supply lines. This applies to any supply lines, not just the ones you have been assigned to work on. Employees who work on energized lines must consider the effects of their actions and account for their own safety as well as the safety of other employees on the job site. This includes simple things, like not bringing a travel mug up in a bucket with you when you are working. If you were to drop something like this from 30 or 40 feet in the air, you could create a hazard for others on the ground.

Employees cannot take conductive objects closer to energized parts than the gap that is allowed by the approach distances outlined in

Tables 441-1 through 441-4. Even if you think lines should be de-energized, you need to consider equipment and lines energized unless you are positive that no current is present. This applies to underground lines as well. You also need to assume that ungrounded metal parts are energized at the highest voltage to which they are exposed. This means that before you start working on any lines or equipment, you need to determine the operating voltage for them.

As with any other type of electrical worker, power line employees must use PPE that is appropriate for the work conditions, equipment, and devices involved in the task that they need to perform. Climbers must use fall protection systems if they will be working more than 10 feet off the ground.

If you will be working from a wooden ladder, do not reinforce it with metal of any kind.

Another aspect of work that you need to be mindful of is working underground. When working in a manhole, you need to test for combustible or flammable gases before entering and NEVER ever smoke in a manhole. Besides the potential for explosions from residual or trapped gasses, cigarette smoke will diminish the oxygen supply.

APPROACH SAFETY

Section 44 provides additional safety rules for supply employees. For example, communication line workers must adhere to a minimum approach distance of 2 feet 2 inches to a 12.47/7.2 kV line. There is a 40-inch clearance requirement between a power supply line and a communication line. If this clearance does not exist on a pole, then a communication line worker would have to call a trained supply employee to perform the communication line work.

Other workers, such as roofers, painters, or chimney sweeps, working in the vicinity of a power line must maintain a minimum 10-foot clearance from any supply line. This may be something that they are completely unaware of, and so, based on Section 42, it becomes your responsibility to inform them of the clearance requirement.

Approach distances when working from a pole or bucket include both an electrical component and an inadvertent movement consideration. For voltages up to 0.750 kV, the inadvertent movement component is the electrical component plus 1 foot. For voltages between 0.751 kV and 72.5 kV, the consideration is the electrical component plus 2 feet. Protective clothing also needs to be rated to accommodate the voltage of the circuits you will be working around. If you are working on a line with a voltage between 51 and 300 V, you must wear cover-alls that are rated for the phase-to-phase or phase-to-ground voltage of the circuit, depending on the exposure of the circuit (Figure 8.7).

Support Structure Clearances

Supply lines are not the only installation elements that have clearance requirements. There are specific distance rules from the supporting structure to a variety of other interferences. For example, a grounded

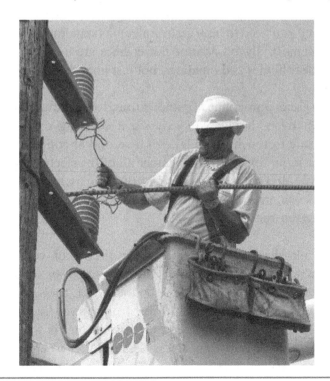

Figure 8.7 Line workers are required to adhere to approach minimums and inadvertent movement allowances.

streetlight pole must provide 15 feet of clearance from the bottom of the grounded luminaire to the top surface of a road or street that is subject to truck traffic. If a supporting structure is up to 15 feet above the road surface it cannot be installed less than 6 inches behind the street side of a redirectional curb and it must be behind a swale-type curb.

Clearances for "pedestrian-only" areas are 14 feet 5 inches, 12 inches, and 9 feet 5 inches consecutively. But be careful using these lower sag limits in locations such as rural or forested areas accessible to horseback riding because then the pedestrian-only criteria will not be met.

Power line safety for electricians

Power supply and communication line workers are not the only people who find themselves exposed to high power voltage hazards. As a commercial or residential electrician you may be exposed to power line risks at their worst and you need to have an overall understanding of how to react. First and foremost, always assume power lines are live. This applies to power lines near homes and buildings, not just lines on poles (Figure 8.8).

Not all energized power lines bounce around the ground sparking or starting fires. Even though you may see a covering on a line, never assume it is safe to touch. All it takes is a second of contact with power lines to cause injury or death. Remember all of the electrical hazards we have already addressed, such as the fact that electricity will cause your muscles to clench, making it impossible to break free from contact with a high voltage current.

Never setup a ladder near power lines. As an electrician, you do not necessarily know what the safe clearances are around power supplies. When you do have to work from a ladder, keep the ladder, tools, and anything else you may be carrying at least 10 feet from power lines. Sometimes you may need to work higher than a ladder and that is when you need to stop first and look for power lines. Use a spotter to ensure that you are complying with safe line clearances. Keep all cranes, scaffolding, and high reach equipment away from supply lines so that you can avoid accidental contact that will cause serious burns or electrocution (Figure 8.9).

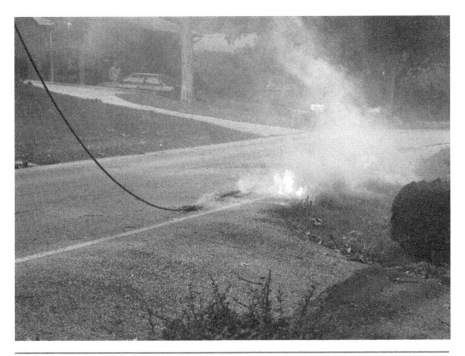

Figure 8.8 Downed power lines that are still energized can spark and cause fires. It is easy to tell that this line is still energized.

When you are performing any construction activities, keep equipment at least 10 feet from power lines and 25 feet from transmission tower lines. Do not climb or trim trees that are close to power lines, and NEVER try to dislodge or knock down a broken tree limb that is stuck on a power line. Maybe that sounds like a no-brainer, but just recently an electrician was electrocuted when he tried to pull a broken tree branch off the power line running to a house he was working on.

The power company in the area where I live runs periodic television ads warning everyone to stay away from fallen power lines. Their motto is "No line is safe to touch, ever." Remember that the earth around a downed line can be energized, so stay away from fallen power lines and be especially careful to avoid metal objects in the area such as street signs, metal handrails, guardrails, or fences that may have become electrified. Because you cannot tell by looking at a fallen power whether it energized or not, it is imperative that you call your local utility right away and report the location of any downed wires. If a line falls on

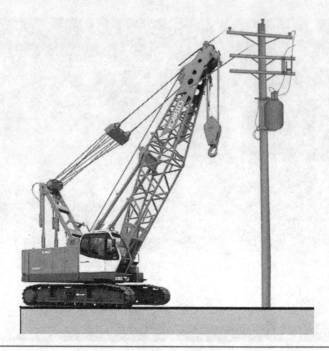

Figure 8.9 Any equipment that extends above the ground, such as cranes, booms, scaffolding, or ladders can accidentally come in contact with high-voltage lines if you do not take distance requirements into consideration.

your car, stay in your car. There is no guarantee that you can safely get out of the car without accidentally touching any part of the car and the ground at the same time (Figure 8.10).

If you have to dig anywhere, for any reason, call your local underground utility locating service first. By law, most states require you to call your local utility to identify any gas, electric, telephone, or other utility lines before you dig. Last year, a nationwide 8-1-1 Call Before You Dig number went into operation. You can't assume that supply cables run underground from a pole to a building service in a straight line. Whether you only have to dig a shallow trench or need to dig down several feet next to a building foundation, any contact you make with a shovel, pick, or other piece of equipment can result in injury or death.

Communication workers know that it is not just power lines that can injure you. Fiber optic cables are becoming a lot more common in most

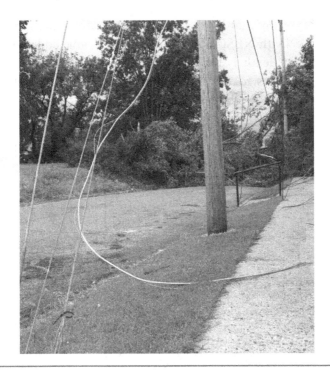

Figure 8.10 Sometimes fallen power lines appear to be harmless and de-energized because no arcs are occurring, when in fact they are energizing the ground and any other metal objects around them.

areas. They're used by phone companies, cable companies, and others utilities for communications purposes. Like power lines, these cables can be broken or knocked down by storms or accidents, but many people assume they don't carry enough current to cause any harm. What fiber optic lines do carry is laser-like light beams that can cause severe eye damage if someone looks into the end of the cable. And the cable strands are made of extremely fine threads of glass, which can easily cut through clothing and skin. Fiber optic cables are usually from ¼ to ¾ inch in diameter, with black insulation, and have multi-colored plastic buffer tubes inside, lined with glass threads, with an outside insulation that often has orange identifying bands or markings.

Whether you are a basic electrician or a power line worker, your safety is contingent on identifying potential high voltage hazards. As a line worker, you are equally responsible for protecting the public and property by ensuring that any installation or maintenance you perform is in compliance with NESC and any other applicable codes. The risk of serious injury or death is far too great to claim ignorance or imprudence when it comes to working around high voltage systems, equipment, and structures (Figure 8.00).

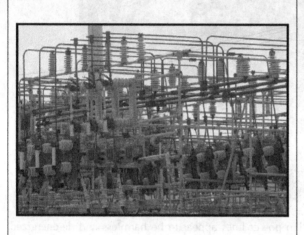

HIGH VOLTAGE

SAFETY

FACTS

The International Electrotechnical Commission defines High Voltage circuits as those with more than 1000 volts for alternating current and at least 1500 V for direct current,
Switchgear line-ups and high-energy arc sources are commonly present in electric power utility substations and generating stations. NFPA 70E should be used to evaluate and calculate potential arc flash hazards and select appropriate PPE
Metal ladders, farm equipment, boat masts, construction machinery, aerial antennas, and similar objects are frequently involved in fatal contact with overhead wires
A tree can become electrified when branches contact high voltage lines
Never burn brush or build fires under power lines because the heat and flames can damage or destroy the wires, insulators and supports of the transmission line;
Many states, such as Georgia, Virginia, Delaware, and Maryland have issued independent High Voltage Safety Acts designed to in work or activity in the vicinity of overhead high voltage lines.
If High Voltage power lines are so dangerous, why can a bird land on the line and not get electrocuted? A bird can sit on a high-voltage wire without harm, since both of its feet are at the same voltage and the bird is not grounded (in contact with the earth)

Figure 8.00 Know the facts of potential hazards when working near high voltage systems.

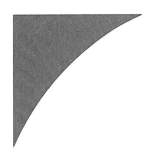

NEC Standards of Safety

Chapter 9

Chapter Outline

189

As an electrician, you are responsible for the health and safety of both yourself and the public. Many people think of NEC requirements as a performance standard, when they actually provide the bare minimum for safe installations. The guidelines are not meant to provide the most convenient or efficient installations and don't even guarantee good service or allow for future expansion. They are designed to provide a standard for safety that protects against electrical shock and thermal effects, as well as dangerous overcurrents, fault currents, and overvoltage.

Conductor sizing

The insulation on a conductor imprisons the dangerous electrical current running through it and guards against shock, fire, and arc incidents. For this reason, you must size conductors properly so that excessive loads do no overheat the conductors and damage the protective insulation. Article 310 of the NEC deals with the minimum size requirements for conductors based on their voltage rating as illustrated in Figure 9.1.

NEC Article 310.15 addresses ampacity, which needs to be cross-referenced to NEC Table 310.5, because Article 310.15 doesn't take voltage drop into consideration. When you run calculations from the tables, you might come up with more than one ampacity, in which case you have to use the lower of two or more ampacities. Additionally, you have to adjust or "derate" your ampacity calculations based on ambient temperature or more than three current-carrying conductors in a wireway. The conductor ampacity that you adjusted from the ambient temperature de-ration calculation has to be multiplied by the percentage of ampacity de-ration that is required by NEC 310.15(B)(2)a (Figure 9.2).

CONDUCTOR AND LOAD SUMMARY

- **Step 1:** Size the overcurrent protection device in accordance with Sections 210.20(A), 215.3, and 384.16(D). These three NEC rules require that the breaker or fuse overcurrent protection device be sized at no less than 100% of the noncontinuous load, plus 125% of the continuous load.

  NOTE: Section 240.6(A) contains the list of standard size overcurrent protection devices.

- **Step 2:** Select the proper conductor size in accordance with Sections 110.4(C), and also NEC 210.19(A), 215.2, and 230.42(A) which required that the conductor be sized no less than 100% of the noncontinuous load, plus 125% of the continuous load. In addition, Section 110.14(C) required you to consider the temperature rating of the equipment terminals when you size the conductors. In order to do this, you need to size the circuit conductors according to the 60°C column of Table 310-16 for equipment that is rated 100 amperes and less. Equipment rated over 100 amperes needs be sized based on the 75°C column of Table 310-16.

- **Step 3:** Now that you have selected the proper conductors to use, you have to protect them against overcurrent in accordance with NEC 240.3, which requires the branch circuit, feeder, and service conductors be protected in accordance with their ampacities as specified in Table 310.16. Remember when you do this, that section 240.3(B) allows you to use the next size up if the conductors are not part of a multi-outlet branch circuit that supplies receptacles, and as long as the ampacity of the conductors doesn't correspond with the standard ampere rating of a overcurrent protection fuse or a circuit breaker listed in NEC 240.6(A). Also, the next higher standard rating can not exceed 800 amperes.

Assume you have 19 kVA of nonlinear loads with 75°C terminals, and that the branch-circuit is supplied by a 208/120 volt, 4-wire, 3-phase. Let's walk through the steps to determine what size branch-circuit overcurrent protection device and conductor (THHN) is required for this installation based on the process we just reviewed.

- ✓ **Step 1:** *Size the overcurrent protection device in accordance with 210.20(A) and 384.16(D).* The first thing that you need to do is to convert the nonlinear load from kVA to amperes:

Amperes = VA/(Volts × 1.732), Amperes = 19,000/(208 volts × 1.732), Amperes = 52.74 amperes. Round up 53 amperes

  The branch-circuit overcurrent protection device has to be sized based on at least 125% of the 53 amperes.

  <u>53 amperes × 125% = 66 amperes*</u>

  *You need a minimum **70 ampere** overcurrent protection device, based on NEC 240.6(A).

- ✓ **Step 2:** *Select the proper conductor size in accordance with Sections 110.4(C), and also NEC 210.19(A), 215.2, and 230.42(A).* NEC 210.19(A) also requires that the branch-circuit conductor be sized no less than 125% of the continuous load.

Figure 9.1—Cont'd

53 amperes × 125% = 66 amperes

You need to pick the conductor based on the 75°C terminals temperature rating of the equipment terminals. No. 6 THHN has a rating of 65 amperes at 75°C, so you can not use that size. You need to go to the next size up.

Use #4 THHN which has a rating of 85 amperes at 75°C.

✓ **Step 3:** Protect the #4 THHN conductor against overcurrent in accordance with NEC 240.3. First, you need to confirm that the #4 THHN is properly protected against overcurrent by the 70 ampere overcurrent protection device listed. To do this, you need to look at the fact that you have a 4-wire, 3-phase service. Since that are more than three current-carrying conductors in the same raceway, you have to adjust the #4 THHN conductor ampacity to the amperage listed in the 90°C column of NEC Table 310.16.

Corrected Ampacity for #4 THHN = Ampacity × Note 8(A). The Adjustment Factor Corrected Ampacity of #4 THHN = 95 amperes × 80%.

Corrected Ampacity #4 THHN = 76 amperes

For the #4THHN that is rated at 76 amperes after ampacity factors, the proper overcurrent protection device will need to be rated at 70 amps in order to comply with the general requirements of NEC 240.3.

Let's work through another example using a 184 amp feeder continuous load on a panelboard with 75°C terminals that supplies nonlinear loads. We will assume that the feeder is supplied by a 4-wire, 3-phase, wye connected system and determine what size feeder overcurrent protection device and THHN conductor are required to meet code standards.

- **Step 1:** Size the overcurrent protection device in accordance with NEC 215.3 and 384-16(D). The feeder overcurrent protection device be sized at least 125% of the184 amperes.

184 amperes × 125% = 230 amperes.

NOTE: According to NEC 240.6(A) you must use a minimum **250 ampere overcurrent protection device**.

- **Step 2:** Select the conductor that will comply with NEC 110.14(C) and with NEC 215.2 which requires the feeder conductor to be sized no less than 125% of the continuous load.

184 amperes × 125% = 230 amperes. You then need to select a conductor according to the 75°C temperature rating of the panelboards terminals.

#4/0 THHN has a rating of 230 amperes at 75°C.

- **Step 3:** Protect the #4/0 conductor against overcurrent based on the requirements in NEC 240.3. Start by verifying that the #4/0 THHN conductor would be adequately protected by a 250 amp overcurrent protection device. Since our

Figure 9.1—Cont'd

sample installation is a 4-wire, 3-phase, wye connected system, you know you will have more than three current-carrying conductors in the same raceway, so you have to correct the #4/0 THHN conductor ampacity by the 90°C column of NEC Table 310-16.

Corrected Ampacity for #4/0 THHN = Ampacity × Note 8(A). The Adjustment Factor Corrected Ampacity for #4/0 THHN = 260 amperes × 80%

Corrected Ampacity for #4/0 THHN = 208 amperes

The #4/0 THHN that is rated at 208 amps after you applied the ampacity correction would not be properly protected by a 250 amp overcurrent protection device, because "the next size up rule" in NEC 240.3(B) would only permit a 225 amp OCPD on your 208 amp conductor. This means you have to increase the conductor size to 250 kcmil in order to comply with the overcurrent protection rules of NEC 240.3

Figure 9.1—Cont'd   Minimum conductor sizes permitted in NEC 310.5.

Number of Current-Carrying Conductors	Values in NEC Tables 310.16 - 310.19 Adjusted for Ambient Temperature, if Necessary
4-6	80 %
7-9	70 %
10-20	50 %
21-30	45 %
31-40	40 %
40 and above	35 %

Figure 9.2   Adjustment factors are required for more than three current-carrying conductors in a raceway or cable.

Here is an example of applying these requirements:

■ Assume you plan on running a *#8 AWG TW copper* conductor in an attic that has an approximate *average ambient temperature of 130°F*. There will be a total of *26 current-carrying conductors* in the conduit.

■ *STEP 1:* Begin by looking at NEC Table 310.16 in the first column (for 60 °C/140°F). You will see that #8 copper TW is rated at 40 A.

- *STEP 2:* In order to determine what correction factor to use, you will need to convert 130°F to centigrade. The formula for this is: C = (F−32) ÷ 9 × 5.

So using this formula, your conversion would work like this:

$$130 - 32 = 98 \quad 98 \div 9 = 10.888 \quad 10.9 \times 5 = 54.5$$

- *STEP 3:* Locate 55 °C in the ambient temperature column of the correction factors section of Table 310.16. You will see that the corresponding correction factor is 0.41.

- *STEP 4:* Multiply the 40 A from Step 1 by the 41% correction factor in Step 3, which will give you a total of 16.4. This means you have 16.4 A of ampacity after the temperature de-ration calculation.

- *STEP 5:* Next, you need to turn back to NEC Table 310.15 (B)(2) and locate the number of current-carrying conductors in your raceway, which we listed in the essential installation information as 26 conductors, and find the adjustment value for ambient temperature that correlates to the quantity of conductors. For between 21 and 30 conductors, you will use the value of 45%.

- *STEP 6:* Next, take the amps you calculated in Step 4 of 16.4 and multiply that times the 45% value you came up with in Step 6: 16.4 × 0.45 = 7.38. This means that 7.38 is the total reduction of ampacity after the ambient temperature de-ration and de-ration for the quantity of conductors are factored in. Round this amperage DOWN and you have 7 A as the true adjusted total ampacity rating of the #8 AWG TS copper conductor.

- *STEP 7:* The NEC requires you to have a minimum ampacity of 15 A for any conductor that is used in a wiring system of 120 V or more (NEC Table 210.3). Furthermore, the conductor must have an ampacity that is no less than the maximum load to be served, based on the requirements of NEC 210.19(A)1.

You just ran all of these calculations only to find that the #8 AWG TW conductor you planned to use in this installation is not permitted for this use. Not only is it not rated at the minimum required 15 A, but because it is smaller than 15 A it is too small to carry the 120-volt service load.

Branch circuit sizing

Branch circuits are the section of a wiring circuit between the final set of fuses or final breaker and the outlets it supplies. Dwelling units require branch circuits with voltages that do not exceed 120 V nominal, and if the circuits are for luminaires or cord-and-plug connected loads don't exceed 1440 V A, or less than ¼ horsepower (Figure 9.3).

NEC Article 210.11 provides the number of branch circuits permitted in any given system and explains that a load that is computed on a VA/area basis has to be evenly proportioned. A wiring system, including the branch circuit panelboard, has to be proportioned to serve the calculated loads and can never exceed the maximums which are specified in NEC 220. Loads must also be evenly proportioned and distributed among the multi-outlet branch circuits with a panelboard. Branch circuit overcurrent protection devices (OCPD) and circuits only have to be installed to serve connected loads. Branch circuit OCPD must have an ampacity of no less than 125% of the continuous loads, plus 100% of the noncontinuous loads.

There are three categories of branch circuit requirements in NEC 210 for dwelling units. The first is the small appliance branch circuit regulation that requires two or more 20-amp small appliance branch circuit outlets. The next is laundry branch circuits, which must have one

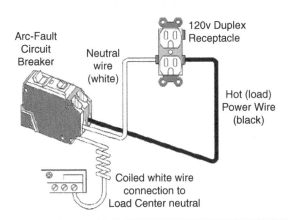

Figure 9.3 A single-pole branch circuit wiring example.

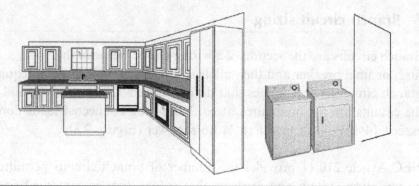

Figure 9.4 Small-appliance and laundry circuits must be included in load calculations.

20-amp branch circuit that does not supply any other outlets and supplies just a laundry receptacle. The third requirement is that there must be a 20-amp branch circuit in any bathroom and that the circuit does not supply any other receptacle (Figure 9.4).

AFCI PROTECTION

Arc-fault circuit interrupter protection is outlined in NEC 210.12. You need to understand that AFCI is not the same as GFCI, even though there are combination units available. The function of an AFCI, which operates at 30 mA, is to protect equipment while a GFCI, which operates at between 4 and 6 mA, is designed to protect people. An AFCI provides protection against the effects of arc faults because it identifies the unique characteristics of arcing and will de-energize a circuit when an arc fault is detected. Any of the 15 or 20 A, 120 V, single-phase branch circuits in a dwelling unit bedroom must have AFCI protection. The 2008 edition of the NEC allows the AFCI device to be located any distance from the panelboard, so long as required wiring methods are used to protect the AFCI device against physical damage. Additionally, the code requires that all 15 and 20 A branch circuits installed in dwelling units have arc-fault circuit interrupter protection (Figure 9.5).

The new clarification in the 2008 NEC 210.12 spells out locations that require AFCI-protection requirements for branch circuits that supply outlets in dwelling unit family rooms, dining rooms, living rooms, parlors, libraries, dens, bedrooms, sunrooms, recreation rooms, closets,

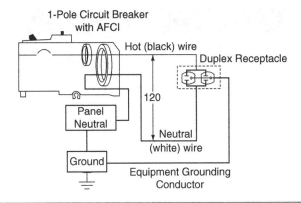

Figure 9.5 An AFCI wiring diagram.

hallways, or similar areas. However, it is important to note that this 120-volt circuit limitation means AFCI protection isn't required for equipment such as baseboard heaters or room air conditioners that are rated at 230 V.

NEC 210.12. Arc-Fault Circuit-Interrupter Protection states that an AFCI provides "protection from the effects of arc faults by recognizing characteristics unique to arcing and by functioning to de-energize the circuit when an arc fault is detected." It is not a GFCI, though combination units do exist. The purpose of an AFCI (30 mA) is to protect equipment. The purpose of a GFCI (4-6 mA) is to protect people.

CIRCUIT RATING

NEC 210.19 provides the rules for minimum amperages and sizes of conductors. One of the key points that you need to be sure you understand is that before you apply any adjustments or correction factors, branch conductors must have an allowable amperage that is not lower than the noncontinuous load of the circuit *plus* 125% of the continuous load. Table 210.21(B)(2) illustrates that the maximum load on any given circuit is 80% of the receptacle rating and circuit rating. You might find it easiest to read the table from right to left because then you will be identifying the load you need to supply first and the circuit rating you need to provide afterwards. Looking at the table in this way, you can see that if you need to supply a 20-amp load, you need to

Maximum Load In Amps	Receptacle Rating In Amps	Circuit Rating In Amps
12	15	15 or 20
16	20	20
24	30	30

Maximum Cord-and-Plug Connected Load to a Receptacle

Figure 9.6 Maximum loads by circuit rating.

install at least a 30-amp receptacle on a 30-amp circuit. An example of the table information is listed in Figure 9.6.

The next rating table in NEC 210.21(B)(3) lists the various sizes of circuits connected to a receptacle. Receptacle ratings for branch circuits that supply two or more receptacles have to fall within the values shown in the table. If the receptacle rating is more than 50 A, then the receptacle cannot be rated less than half of the branch circuit rating (Figure 9.7).

The total rating of utilization equipment fastened in place, with the exception of light fixtures, cannot exceed 50% of the branch-circuit amperage rating when lighting units, cord-and-plug connected equipment that isn't fastened in place, or both of these are also supplied. The safety rationale behind this is to prevent a circuit overload when an additional load is added, for example if someone plugs in a vacuum cleaner. The solution is to separate circuits by putting lights on one circuit, dedicated loads (fastened in place) on different circuits, and convenience receptacles on separate circuits.

Place lights on separate circuits, dedicated (fastened in place) loads on separate circuits, and convenience receptacles on separate circuits.

Receptacle Rating In Amps		Circuit Rating In Amps
15	⇨	15 or 20
20	⇨	20
30	⇨	30

Receptacle Ratings for Associated Circuit Sizes

Figure 9.7 Receptacles for branch circuits.

Cord-and-plug connected equipment that is not fastened in place, such as a table saw for example, cannot have an amperage rating that is more than 80% of the branch-circuit rating. Portable equipment, like a hair dryer, may have a UL listing up to 100% of the circuit rating, but you have to remember that the NEC is an installation standard, not a product standard. As an electrician, you have no way of knowing if a circuit will be used at 80% of the branch-circuit rating, but you must install to that standard.

To keep things simple when you are sizing conductors for branch circuits, remember that the OCPD defines the circuit. If a 20-amp circuit contains 8 AWG conductors because of voltage drop, it is still a 20 A circuit. The rating of the branch circuit is determined by the size of the OCPD. An individual receptacle on a single branch circuit cannot have an amperage that is less than the rating of the OCPD, as specified in NEC Article 210.21(B)(1). Also remember that a single receptacle has only one contact device on its yoke as described in Article 100, which means that you would treat a duplex receptacle as two receptacles.

Everything you need to know on a regular basis about branch circuit requirements is summarized in NEC Table 210.24. Simply look for the circuit rating, which is based on the load you need to supply, and the table indicates the minimum conductor and tap sizes, overcurrent protection, and maximum load. It also lists which lamp holders are permitted and the required receptacle rating.

Feeder sizing

The definition of a feeder is the circuit conductors that supply power to a branch-circuit overcurrent device or to a panel that contains the OCPD. The power can come from the service equipment, a separately derived system, or other power supply source. So, what is the main difference between a branch circuit and a feeder? A feeder runs between an OCPD at the supply and a downstream OCPD typically supplying a branch circuit. On the other hand, a branch circuit runs between the OCPD and an outlet, which is considered the final load. In other words, a feeder supplies power to a branch-circuit OCPD and that OCPD, in turn, powers the branch circuit. You need to remember that you don't size that branch circuit OCPD based on feeder calculations, but rather on the branch-circuit load calculations and receptacle outlet requirements. NEC Article 215 is fairly short because it only outlines the rules for installation, minimum size, and ampacity of feeders.

If your computations result in a fraction of an ampere that is less than 0.5, you are permitted to drop the fraction. This is because you are just calculating here, not selecting components, which are available only in standard sizes. The various safety factors in the code already account for enough headroom that dropping a fraction of an amp won't matter.

When you calculate feeder-circuit conductor loads, the minimum size, before any adjustments or correction factors are applied, needs to be no less than the non-continuous load *plus* 125% of the continuous load. If the feeder conductors carry the total load supplied by service conductors that are 55 A or less, then the feeder conductor amperage cannot be less than the service conductor amperage. To size feeders that supply transformers, you need to add the transformer nameplate ratings together and make sure that the feeder conductor amperage is not less than that sum.

THINK BACKWARDS AND FORWARDS: As you run calculations as they are laid out in NEC Article 220, keep in mind that these are used in conjunction with provisions from other articles. Results from calculations in Parts III, IV, and V of Article 220, for example, are used with the provision in 215.2(A)(1) to find the minimum feeder-circuit conductor size. The calculations in NEC 220 are also necessary in determining the minimum fuse or breaker size allowed for feeders as required by NEC 215.3.

To protect feeder circuits, you must install overcurrent protection. If a feeder supplies a continuous load, or a combination of continuous and non-continuous loads, then the OCPD cannot be rated any less than the non-continuous load plus 125% of the continuous load amperage. Both of the rating requirements have an exception for assemblies that are listed to operate at 100% of their ratings, including the OCPD. In these cases, the ratings can be equal to the sum of the continuous and non-continuous loads.

A common neutral is permissible for two sets of four-wire or five-wire feeders, as well as for two or three sets of three-wire feeders. Grounding is required for all feeders that supply branch circuits that require equipment grounding conductors. You can tap two-wire DC circuits or AC circuits with two or more ungrounded conductors. In this situation you would tap from the ungrounded conductors of the circuits that have a grounded neutral conductor and use switching devices in each tapped circuit that have a pole in each ungrounded conductor. The grounded conductor of a feeder circuit must follow the same standards of identification as any grounded conductor, which means it must have a continuous white or gray outer insulated covering or three continuous white stripes on an insulated covering that is not green. Equipment grounding conductors need to be identified in accordance with NEC 250.119.

NFPA 70E also addresses current-carrying conductors, buses, switches, and disconnects, and requires that they be maintained to conduct rated current without overheating and to withstand available fault current.

One of the most important aspects of planning a safe electrical installation is running accurate load calculations. There are a couple of things to keep in mind when you are running these computations. First of all, load calculations are affected by demand factors, which is the ratio of the maximum demand of a system to the total connected load of that system. While different loads have different demand factors, the demand factor is always equal to or less than one. Safe and compliant installations depend of your ability to achieve accurate calculation results. Let's walk through the process, beginning with common receptacles.

The computed load of a feeder or service cannot be less than the sum of computed loads on the branch circuits. You do not select the feeder or service breakers based on the sum of the branch breaker ratings. You select them based on the total load supplied by that feeder or service. That total load must account for demand factors and diversity factors (for example, you don't run your air conditioner and heater at the same time, and you wouldn't be using all 19 welding receptacles in a small shop at one time) and other items detailed elsewhere in Article 220. NEC Table 220.11 lists the demand factors for lighting loads in various types of occupancies. This is not the reference you use to determine the quantity of branch circuits for general illumination.

GENERAL USE RECEPTACLES

All general-use receptacle outlets that are rated at either 15 or 20 A installed in dwellings are included as a part of the general lighting-load calculations. Let's look at an example. Assuming that a living room in a single-family home is 13 feet × 15 feet, first you have to space the receptacle installation in accordance with NEC 210.52 (Figure 9.8).

Because of the room's dimensions, nine receptacle outlets are required. Unlike receptacles for non-dwelling installations that must be calculated at 180 V A each, dwelling receptacles do not require any additional load. The general lighting load for this room would need to be calculated in accordance with 220.12 and Table 220.12, which would be 3 V A per square foot. For a 13 feet × 15 feet living room, this equates to 195 square feet times 3 V A, for a total 585 Units. The next step in the calculation process is not spelled out in the code article. Based on a normal residential service size of 120/240 V, you need to complete the calculation by dividing the unit total by 120 (V). This results in 4.875 (585/120 = 4.875), which should be rounded up to 5.

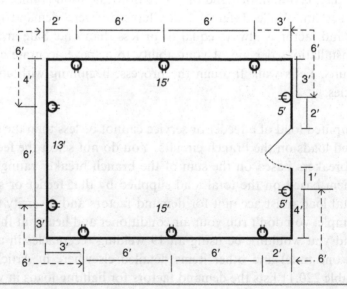

Figure 9.8 Living room receptacle requirements.

The load calculation formula does not change when the number of receptacle outlets, specified in 220.14(J)(1) through (J)(3), is more than the required minimum.

Load calculation does not vary, even if you add more outlets for a space than are required by the standard. Going back to our 13 feet × 15 feet living room example, if you added twice as many receptacles, the load for space would be calculated exactly the same as in our example: 195 square feet × 3 = 585/120 = 4.875, which still rounds up to 5.

CALCULATING BRANCH CIRCUITS

To determine the minimum number of 15-amp and 20-amp branch circuits needed in dwellings for lighting and general-use outlets, you need to start with the floor area again. Begin by determining the square footage of the space and then, using Table 220.12, find the general lighting load required. The resulting lighting load is in amps, which needs to be divided by either 15 or 20 A for the branch circuits. Let's look at a new example. Assume you have a single-family home with outside dimensions of 50 feet by 30 feet.

- *STEP 1:* Determine the square footage of the dwelling by multiplying the length time the width: 50 feet × 30 feet = 1500 square feet.

- *STEP 2:* Calculate the general light load using Table 220.12, which indicates that the unit load for a dwelling unit is 3 V A per square foot. So, you would multiply 1500 sq ft × 3 = 4500 V A.

- *STEP 3:* Confirm that the dwelling voltage is 120/240 V and divide the minimum light load that you calculated in Step 2 by 120 V: 4500/120 = 37.5 which should be rounded up to 38.

- *STEP 4:* Now, to determine the minimum number of 15-amp, two-wire circuits that are required by the code, you need to divide the load you determined in Step 3 by 15 A. This comes out to 38 divided by 15 which equals 2533, which needs to be rounded up to 3. Now you have determined that at least three 15 A, two-wire circuits are required for your 50 feet × 30 feet dwelling installation.

To calculate the minimum number of 20-amp general-purpose branch circuits, you use 20 as your factor in Step 14 instead of 15. So the calculation process ends up looking like this:

- 50 feet × 30 feet = 1500 sq feet

- 1500 sq feet × 3 = 4500 V A

- 4500/120 = 37.5 (round up to 38)

- 38 divided by *20* = 1.9 which needs to be rounded up to 2

So, based on our sample, the minimum number of 20-amp, two-wire branch circuits required for our dwelling is two. But wait, there's more. You need to have at least one 20-amp laundry circuit and a minimum of two 20-amp small appliance branch circuits to meet code requirements, even though your minimum load calculation resulted in only two. Think about any other associated code requirements that you may need to consider. For example, bathroom branch circuits that supply receptacle outlets also must be rated at 20 A. However, no additional load calculation is required for the bathroom circuits, so you still only need three.

Feeder and service loads

Understanding how to perform load calculations is an important part of an electrician's professional career and critical for hazard-free installations. Feeder and service load calculations include demand factors that should be applied to some of the branch-circuit load calculations that you have already run. NEC Annex D is made up of numerous examples intended to explain how to calculate loads based on actual examples of various conditions such as multifamily dwellings and industrial feeders in a common raceway.

GENERAL LIGHTING LOADS

You can actually lower the calculated lighting load of a feeder or service by utilizing the lighting load demand factors for certain occupancy types. NEC Table 220.42 lists the demand factors that apply to the portion of the total branch circuit load calculated for general lighting (illumination). Four types of occupancy lighting load conditions are provided: single-family and multifamily dwelling units, hospitals, hotels and motels, and storage warehouses. The hotel and motel standard includes apartment or rooming houses that do not have provisions for cooking by the tenants.

> General lighting loads are based on the square footage (or square meter) of the occupancy space and the calculation factors only vary based on the type of occupancy.

Let's look at a single-family home with a calculated floor area of 4000 square feet as an example of how to apply these demand factors. The portion of the lighting load that is calculated at 100% is first 3000 V A or less. The demand factor is 35% for the portion of the lighting load that ranges between 3001 and 120,000 V A. Next, we have to go through the process of calculating the comprehensive general lighting load by using all of the code requirements and this table to apply demand factors for our 4000 square foot home.

- *STEP 1:* Since you know the total floor area, begin by multiplying the square footage of 4000 by the 3 V A per square foot required in NEC Table 220.12: 4000 × 3 = 12,000. This is the base general lighting load.

- *STEP 2:* Next, we need to add the minimum of a single laundry circuit and two small appliance circuits that we know are required for a single-family dwelling—this was discussed in the section on NEC 210.11 in the previous chapter. Now that we have looked backwards, we have to read ahead to the circuit load requirements in NEC 220.52. Here we see that we must use 1500 V A for each two-wire, small appliance branch circuit. So we multiply 1500 × 2 = 3000.

- *STEP 3:* NEC 220.52(B) requires that we multiply each laundry branch circuit by 1500 V A also, so we need to include another 1500 V A to our calculation.

- *STEP 4:* At this point, let's add together what we have so far:

  - 12,000 (from Step 1) + 3000 (from Step 2) + 1500 (from Step 3) = 16,500

- *STEP 5:* Use this total of 16,500 as your base to run the demand factors. The first 3000 is a straight 100% which is simply 3000 V A.

The remaining 13,500 (16,500-3000 = *13,500*) is subject to the 35% demand: 13,500 × 35% = 4725.

- *STEP 6:* This means that the general lighting load for this one-family dwelling ends up being: 3000 (from Step 1) + 4725 (Step 5) = *7725* V A.

Now you have determined the most basic general lighting load for the house. However, there are additional electrical load elements that can affect service, circuit, and feeder sizing for any installation.

ADDITIONAL SERVICE AND FEEDER LOADS

Any fixed electric space heater loads are calculated at 100% of the total connected load. Under no circumstances can the feeder or service load current ratings be less than the largest supplied branch circuit rating. Whereas motor and motor-compressor loads must be calculated at 125%, fixed electric space heating loads are simply based on 100%, but 100% of what exactly?

Assume you are reviewing plans for a small office and the specifications call for seven wall heaters. Each heater has a rating of 3000 W at 240 V (Figure 9.9).

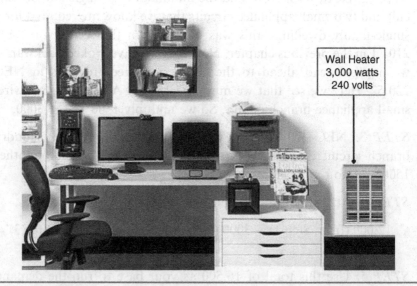

Wall Heater
3,000 watts
240 volts

Figure 9.9 Office heater loads must be based on the total current draw of all the heaters.

How much load will these heaters add to a 240-volt, single-phase service? If you just take NEC 220.51 on face value, then you would calculate the heaters at 100% (7 × 3000 = 21,000 W) and call your formula done. However, we also need to determine the total current draw of the heaters. To do this, divide the total watts you just calculated by the 240 V:

■ 21,000 ÷ 240 = 87.5 Remember to round-up to 88 A

The calculated load for these seven 3000-watt, 240-volt heaters on a 240-volt, single-phase service is 88 A.

This process is fine if you just have standard heating only units. But what if you are installing a heating and cooling combination unit? Heating units that are equipped with blower motors must be calculated in accordance with NEC 220.50 and 220.51. To do this, let's assume we are going to install a heating/cooling package unit in a single-family dwelling. The specs for the unit indicate that the electric heater is rated 9.6 kW and 240 V and the blower motor inside the package unit is a ½ horsepower, 240-volt motor. Your job is to find out how much of a load this combination unit adds to the home's 240-volt, single-phase service. Follow the steps in the process below:

■ *STEP 1:* Convert the 9.6 kW from kilowatts to basic watts. This is from your basic electrical math that you had to learn before you could get your electrician's license. 9.6 × 1000 (kilo) = 9600 W. Since the load needs to be eventually determined in amps, you will need to convert the watts to amps. Using Ohm's Law, this is done by dividing the watts by the amps: 9600 ÷ 240 = 40 A (Figure 9.10).

■ *STEP 2:* Next, you need to determine the full-load current in amperes of the ½ horsepower, single-phase, 240-volt motor. The information on how to do this is located in NEC article 430

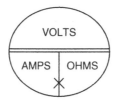

Figure 9.10 Ohms Law diagram.

that focuses on motors, motor circuits, and controllers. NEC Table 430.248 is a simple chart that lists the horsepower of A/C motors running at full-load currents and usual speeds with normal torque characteristics. In other words, the table is geared toward generic, average conditions. The motor we are using in our example is rated at 240 V, but when you look at Table 430.248, you may get a little confused because there is no column for motors rated at 240 V. Just read the description of the table and you will see that the currents listed can be used for 110-120 V and 220-240 V (Figure 9.11).

■ *STEP 3:* Based on Table 430.248, the full-load current for a ½ horsepower, single-phase, 240-volt motor is 4.9 A. Unlike some of the calculations we have done previously, you need to use the exact voltage listed in the table—do NOT round up.

■ *STEP 4:* Since we are starting with watts in Step 1, we need to convert the 4.9 amperage rating to watts.

■ *STEP 5:* Now add the amps from Step 1 to the amps in Step 4: 40 + 4.9 = 44.9 A. This time you do need to round up to 45 A. This means that the total calculated ampere load for our heating and cooling package unit, including the blower motor, on a 240-volt, single-phase service is 45 A.

Keep in mind that unless this unit is the largest motor in the feeder or service load calculation, you do not need to include any additional demand factors. But just for the sake of knowing how to take these calculations to the next level, let's say that our ½ horsepower blower motor is the largest motor we have to include in the calculations for the house service. That being the case, the ampacity cannot be less than 125% of the full-load current rating *plus* the calculated load of the electric heat. Remember that our goal in all of this is to determine how much load all of the various elements in the house wiring layout will

HORSEPOWER	115 VOLTS	200 VOLTS	208 VOLTS	230 VOLTS
1/6	4.4 amps	2.5 amps	2.4 amps	2.2 amps
1/4	5.8 amps	3.3 amps	3.2 amps	2.9 amps
1/3	7.2 amps	4.1 amps	4.0 amps	3.6 amps
1/2	9.8 amps	5.6 amps	5.4 amps	**4.9 amps**

Full-load amperage requirements for electric motors

Figure 9.11 A quick reference electric motor load chart.

add to the dwelling's service requirements. To determine how much load this package unit will add to our 240-volt, single-phase service, we need to multiply the motor's full-load current by 125% before adding it to the electric heat: 4.9 (from Table 430.248, Step 4 above) × 125% = 6.125. Next we have to add in the amps we calculated in Step 1 above of 40 A to arrive at our total amperage: 40 + 6.125 = 46 A. You can see the difference in the calculated load when the blower motor is the largest motor in the service load calculation. It has gone from 45 to 46 A. This 1 A change can be the difference in a service load that is code compliant and one that is not.

FEEDER AND SERVICE LOADS VERSES BRANCH-CIRCUIT LOADS

Although fixed electric space heating loads are calculated in accordance with NEC 220.51 to determine the appropriate feeder and service loads, branch-circuit loads must be calculated in accordance with NEC article 424. By looking at NEC Table 220.3, we know that we have to specifically go to Section 424.3 to find "Fixed Electric Space Heater Equipment, Branch-Circuit Sizing." As previously discussed, branch-circuit conductors must have an ampacity that is not less than 125% of the continuous load. If we use our heating and cooling package unit as an example again, how would we now establish that the minimum size 75 °C branch-circuit conductors are required for the unit?

- *STEP 1:* The service load for this unit was calculated at 100%, but in accordance with NEC 430.22(A), the blower motor also had to be calculated at 125%. We went through this process and came up with a combined blower motor and heating element current of 44.9 A. Now we have to multiply that amperage by 125%: 44.9 × 125% = 56.125 Round this DOWN to 56 A.

- *STEP 2:* We have now established that the 75 °C branch-circuit conductors needed for our heating/cooling package unit must be at least 56 A.

- *STEP 3:* If you wanted to find out the minimum size 75 °C conductors that would be required to feed this heating/cooling package unit, you would need to look in Annex B, Table B310.3 in the back of the code book. Here you will see that for 50 A at 75 °C you can use 8 AWG, but since we need 56 A, we have to jump up to the next level which is 6 AWG copper conductors for use between 51 and 68 A.

No additional calculations are necessary as long as the heating and cooling unit provides minimum circuit ampacity and maximum branch-circuit overcurrent protection that is shown on the nameplate. If our heating and cooling package unit was listed for a minimum/maximum fuse or HACR-type breaker of 100 A on the nameplate then the branch-circuit load would have to be protected by a 100-ampere fuse or HACR-type circuit breaker.

Small Appliance and Laundry Loads

Small-appliance branch-circuit loads must be included in the load calculations in order to determine the approved feeder and service loads for dwelling units. We included them already when we were calculating our comprehensive general lighting loads. NEC 220.52 requires 1500 V A for each two-wire small-appliance branch circuit. Two or more 20-ampere small-appliance branch circuits required by NEC 210.11(C)(1) have to serve all wall and floor receptacle outlets, as well as all of the countertop outlets and all of the receptacle outlets for refrigeration equipment.

If the load is subdivided through two or more feeders, the calculated load for each cannot be less than the 1500 V A for each two-wire small-appliance branch circuit. For example, let's say that a one-family dwelling will have three panelboards, not counting the service equipment. One of the panelboards is going to supply three small-appliance branch circuits and the other two panelboards will not supply any small-appliance branch circuits. We have to multiply the three small appliance branch circuits by the required 1500 A: $3 \times 1500 = 4500$. This means that 4500 A must be included when we calculate the load for the panelboard with the three small-appliance branch circuits. But, since the other two panelboards don't supply any small-appliance branch circuits, we will not include these loads in our calculations.

When you are looking at small-appliance circuits, remember that not all circuits in a kitchen are required to have 20 A circuits. Refrigeration equipment can be supplied from an individual branch circuit that is rated at 15 A or more. But, if the refrigeration equipment is not supplied by its own individual branch circuit, then it has to be supplied by a 20 A small-appliance branch circuit, and the load has to be calculated at the same 1500 V A as any of the other small-appliance circuits. The load for laundry circuits is a flat 1500 A and only one circuit has to be provided. Again, you can add more circuits, but you always have to provide at least one.

ELECTRIC CLOTHES DRYER LOADS

The load for each household electric clothes dryer in a dwelling unit has to be the larger of either the nameplate rating or 5000 V A. Unlike the required minimum load of 1500 V A for a laundry branch circuit, there is no required minimum load if an electric clothes dryer is not going to be installed, for example if a gas dryer is going to be installed. When you calculate the load for a feeder or service when an electric clothes dryer will be installed, you have to include a load of at least 5000 V A and one to four dryers is calculated at 100%.

FEEDER AND SERVICE LOAD CALCULATIONS

Dwelling unit feeder and service loads with a connected load that are served by a single 120/240-volt or 208Y/120-volt three-wire service or feeder conductors of 100 A or more must have a total calculated load that is the result of adding the loads formulas in NEC 220.82(B) and 220.82(C). The first step is to take 100% of the first 10 kW and add to it 40% of the following loads:

- 3 V A per square foot of the dwelling unit for the general lighting and general-use receptacles. Remember that the dwelling unit square footage should not include any garages, open porches, or unfinished spaces that will not be finished off in the future.

- 1500 V A for every two-wire, 20 A small appliance branch circuit and laundry branch circuit.

- The nameplate rating of all of the appliances that will be fastened in place or permanently connected, such as ranges, clothes dryers, and water heaters.

- The nameplate amperage or kVA rating of any motors and of any low-power-factor loads.

Next, you need to add the largest of the following kVA loads:

- 100% of any air conditioning/cooling nameplate ratings.

- 100% of any heating nameplate rating if you are installing a heat pump without any supplemental electric heating.

- 100% of the nameplate rating of any heating systems, such as electric thermal storage units, that will have a typical continuous load that will be at the full value listed on the equipment nameplate.

- 100% of any heat pump compressor nameplate rating and 65% of any supplemental central electric space heaters. There is an exemption to this part of the calculation, which is that if the heat pump compressor is installed in a manner that keeps it from operating at the same time as the supplemental heaters then it doesn't have to be added to the heaters as part of the total central heating load.

- 65% of the nameplate rating for any electric space heating if there are less than four individually controlled units.

- 40% of the nameplate rating for any electric space heating if there are four or more separately controlled units.

SERVICE LOADS

The NEC lists two calculation requirements for determining the ampacity of the service-entrance conductors before any adjustment or correction factors are applied. The ampacity cannot be less than:

- The total of all non-continuous loads plus 125% of the continuous loads

- The total of all of the non-continuous loads, plus the continuous load if the service-entrance conductors are terminated in an OCPD that is rated to operate at 100% of the conductor's rating

The service equipment has to be either enclosed or guarded per NEC 230.62 (A)(1) and (A)(2). This means that any energized parts must be enclosed so they cannot be exposed to accidental contact or, if they are not enclosed, they must be installed on a panelboard, switchboard, or control board in a suitable location as described in NEC 110.27.

The service disconnect means cannot be rated at less than the load it would carry, and it can never be rated lower than any of the following:

- 15 A minimum for disconnects to a service for the limited loads of single branch circuits

- 30 A minimum for disconnects to a service for no more than two two-wire branch circuits

- 100 A minimum for disconnects to a single-family dwelling service

- 60 A minimum for all other service disconnect means

There are limited types of equipment which can be connected to the supply side of a service disconnect means, including cable limiters, instrument transformers for current and voltage, impedance shunts, arrestors, and ground-fault protection devices that are installed as part of the equipment that is listed and only if a suitable overcurrent protection and disconnect means is provided. In addition, ground-fault protection of equipment is required to be directly connected to ground for any solidly grounded wye electrical services between 150 V to ground and 600 V phase-to-phase for any service disconnect that is rated at 1000 A or more.

Overcurrent protection

OCPD are meant to protect against the potentially dangerous effects of overcurrents, such as an overload current or a short-circuit current, referred to as fault current. Equipment damage or personal injury or even death can result from the improper application of a device's voltage rating, current rating, or interrupting rating. Something as simple as a circuit breaker can protect against this damage, but if a fuse or circuit breaker doesn't have an adequate voltage rating, it can rupture or explode while attempting to stop fault currents beyond their interrupting ratings.

The OCPD voltage rating is a function of its capacity to open a circuit under overcurrent conditions, and determines the ability of the OCPD to suppress and snuff out the internal arcing that occurs during an overcurrent condition. OCPD can be rated for AC voltage, DC voltage, or both, and often an AC/DC voltage rated OCPD will have an AC

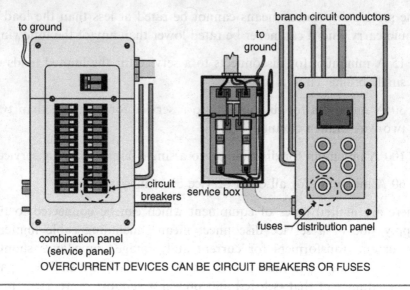

OVERCURRENT DEVICES CAN BE CIRCUIT BREAKERS OR FUSES

Figure 9.12 Typical overcurrent protection devices are either circuit breakers or fuses.

voltage rating that is different from its DC voltage rating. There are two types of AC rated OCPD: straight voltage rated and slash voltage rated. All fuses are straight voltage rated, but some circuit breakers are slash voltage rated at 480/277 V, 240/120 V, or 600/347 V (Figure 9.12).

NEC 240.4(D) establishes conductor size limitation standards. The ampere rating of a fuse or circuit breaker is the maximum amount of current that it can safely carry without opening. The OCPD cannot exceed the following:

- 15 A for 14 AWG

- 20 A for 12 AWG

- 30 A for 10 AWG

- 15 A for 12 AWG and 25 A for 10 AWG aluminum and copper-clad aluminum after any correction factors for ambient temperature and number of conductors have been applied

Standard circuit breaker sizes are listed in Figure 9.13.

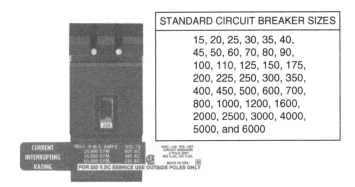

STANDARD CIRCUIT BREAKER SIZES
15, 20, 25, 30, 35, 40, 45, 50, 60, 70, 80, 90, 100, 110, 125, 150, 175, 200, 225, 250, 300, 350, 400, 450, 500, 600, 700, 800, 1000, 1200, 1600, 2000, 2500, 3000, 4000, 5000, and 6000

Figure 9.13 Standard circuit breaker sizes.

Typically, the amperage rating of a fuse or a circuit breaker is based on 125% of the continuous load current. And since conductors are also typically calculated at 125% of the continuous load current, the conductor ampacity wouldn't be exceeded. For example, a 40-amp continuous load conductor multiplied by 125% must be rated to carry 50 A, so a 50-amp circuit breaker is the largest that should be used (Figure 9.14).

There are certain circumstances when you can use a fuse or circuit breaker ampere rating that is greater than the current-carrying capacity of the circuit. A typical example would be motor circuits because dual-element, time-delay fuses are generally allowed to be sized up to 175% or the next standard of the motor full-load amps. Figure 9.15 illustrates a 1.15 SF motor.

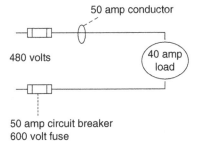

Figure 9.14 Multiplying both the conductor size and the circuit breaker size by 125% protects the circuit ampacity from being exceeded.

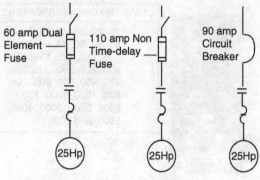

460 volt 3-phase Motor rated @ 25Hp, 34 amps
50 amp Conductor rated for 8 AWG, 75° C

Figure 9.15 This motor circuit would allow fuses sized at exactly 1.75 × 34 A = 59.5 A, requiring the use of the next standard size of 60 A.

GENERATORS

As with other motors, NEC 445.11 requires a generator to have a nameplate giving the manufacturer's name, the rated frequency, power factor, number of AC phases, the subtransient and transient impedances, the rating in kilowatts or kilovolt amperes, a rating for the normal volts and amps, rated revolutions per minute, insulation system class, any rated ambient temperature or temperature rise, and a time rating. The size and type of OCPD will be based on this critical data.

NEC 445.12 defines the basic overcurrent protection standards for various types of generators. A constant-voltage generator must be protected from overloads by either the generator's inherent design or circuit breakers, fuses, or other forms of overcurrent protection that are considered suitable for the conditions of use. This is true except for AC generator exciters (Figure 9.16).

Two-wire, DC generators are allowed to have overcurrent protection in only one conductor if the overcurrent device is triggered by the entire current that is generated other than the current in the shunt field. For this reason, the overcurrent device cannot open the shunt field. If the two-wire generator operates at 65 V or less and is driven by an individual motor then the overcurrent device protection device needs to kick-in

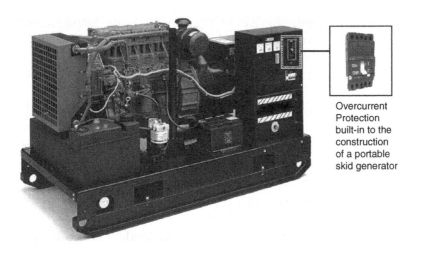

Overcurrent
Protection
built-in to the
construction
of a portable
skid generator

Figure 9.16 All generators must have some form of overcurrent protection.

if the generator is delivering up to 150% of its full-load rated current. When a two-wire DC generator is used in conjunction with balancer sets it accomplishes the neutral points for the three-wire system. This means it requires an overcurrent device that is sized to disconnect the three-wire system if an extreme unbalance occurs in the voltage or current.

For three-wire DC generators, regardless of whether they are compound or shunt wound, one overcurrent device must be installed in each armature lead, and must be connected so that it is activated by the entire current from the armature. These overcurrent devices need to have either a double-pole, double-coil circuit breaker or a four-pole circuit breaker connected in both the main and equalizer leads, plus two more overcurrent devices, one in each armature lead. The OCPD must be interlocked so that no single pole can be opened without simultaneously disconnecting both leads of the armature from the system. The ampacity of the conductors that run from the generator terminals to the first distribution device that contains overcurrent protection cannot be less than 115% of the nameplate current rating for the generator per NEC 445.13.

All generators must be equipped with at least one disconnect that is lockable in the open position that will allow the generator and all of its associated protective devices and controls to be disconnected entirely from the circuits that are supplied by the generator.

TRANSFORMERS

NEC 450 covers the installation requirements for transformers. Transformers have a primary and a secondary voltage. The calculation of the relationship between the primary and secondary voltage is the primary coil voltage divided by the number of turns in the primary equals the total of the secondary coil voltage divided by the number of turns in the wire of the secondary:

$$\frac{\text{Primary coil voltage}}{\#\text{ of turns of wire in the primary}} = \frac{\text{Secondary coil voltage}}{\#\text{ of turns of wire in the secondary}}$$

Let's say you know the incoming, or "primary," voltage to a transformer is going to be 120 V. You also know that the primary has 75 turns and the secondary has 150 turns, but you don't know what the secondary voltage will be. All you have to do is start by dividing the primary volts by the number of primary turns: $120 \div 75 = 1.6$.

Since you know the number of turns in the secondary, you would now multiply the 150 secondary turns by the primary current of 1.6:150 × 1.6 = 240. Now you have determined that the secondary voltage is 240 V.

Transformer overcurrent protection methods are based on the voltage size of the transformer, and the overcurrent device has to be rated or set no more than 125% of the rated full-load input current of the autotransformer. If you run you calculation and the rated input current is 9 A or more, but the size doesn't correspond to the standard rating of a fuse or nonadjustable circuit breaker, you need to use the next higher standard size overcurrent device. If the rated input current of the autotransformer is less than 9 A, an overcurrent device rated or set at not more than 167% of the input current should be used. Overcurrent devices cannot be installed in series with the shunt winding of the autotransformer between points A and B as shown in Figure 9.17.

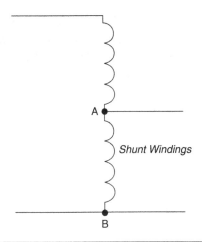

Figure 9.17 Overcurrent devices are prohibited from being installed in series with the shunt winding between points A and B.

Clearance safety

Clearances are specified to protect against heat and fire hazards. For example, an electrical cabinet has to be installed in drywall or plaster so that the front edge of the cabinet doesn't set back farther than 6 inches from the finished surface of the wall. If the cabinet is installed in wood or a combustible material, then it has to be flush with the finished surface.

Anywhere conductors enter the cabinet, there must be adequately closed openings. Conductors in an enclosure for switches or overcurrent devices cannot fill the wiring space by more than 40% of the cross-section area inside the enclosure and they cannot fill the cross-sectional area of the space by more than 75%.

There must be at least 1 inch of airspace between a cabinet door and any live metal parts, including fuses (NEC 312.11(A)(2).

Unused cable or raceway openings in equipment cases, boxes, or auxiliary gutters must be effectively closed to provide the equivalent protection of the wall of the equipment. This also means that conductors in underground or subsurface enclosures that people might need to enter to install or maintain equipment have to be racked. This provides safe and easy access. Also, internal parts of electrical equipment, such as busbars, insulators, or wiring terminals cannot be damaged, bent, broken or cut, or contaminated by materials like paint or plaster, abrasives, or corrosive residues.

Switchboards that are not totally enclosed must have a clearance of 3 feet from the top of the switchboard to a ceiling constructed of wood, drywall, or any other combustible material. Transformers must be readily accessible to qualified personnel for inspection and maintenance per NEC 450.13. Dry-type transformers rated less than 600 V and 112½ kVA must be separated from combustible materials, such as drywall, by a fire-resistant, heat insulating barrier or a minimum of 12 inches of open space. If transformers exceed 112½ kVA, Class 155 then they must be separated by either the fire-resistant barrier or 6 feet horizontally and 12 feet vertically from combustible materials.

ARC WELDING

Welders can encounter major health hazards including fumes and gases, arc rays and sparks, and electric shock. Arc welding uses a welding power supply to create an electric arc between two surfaces or by a heating rod with an electrode until it melts from overcurrent. They can use either DC or AC current, and consumable or non-consumable electrodes. Either method results in a large momentary current draw. NEC Article 630 focuses on adequately sizing the conductors and circuit protection to handle these welding loads. The supply conductors for welders cannot be less than the current values calculated by multiplying the rated primary current in amperes that are shown on the welding machine nameplate by the factor for the machine's duty cycle that is listed in NEC 630-11(A). Each welder must have overcurrent protection rated no less than 200% of the rated primary current of the welder. Because of the safety risks from overheating conductors, welding cable has requirements other conductors don't have. For example, the insulation on these cables must be flame-retardant.

Regardless of the application, conductors and loads must be sized based on the National Electrical Code to guard against hazards. Overcurrent protection, insulation, airspace, and distance from combustible materials all work together to reduce the risk of shock, overheating, and fire damage. When you are installing basic electrical elements, remember that both your safety and the safety of the people and property you are working for are at risk. Since NEC standards are established to ensure installations that are focused on safety, compliance is both mandatory and your best way of reducing your professional and personal risk (Figure 9.00).

CONDUCTOR AND OVERCURRENT PROTECTION SIZING

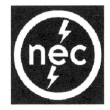

Determine conductor sizing and overcurrent protection based on:

1. Continuous loads
2. Terminal temperature ratings
3. Conductor insulation
4. Conductor ampacity
5. Special application
6. System voltage

Size overcurrent protection devices in accordance with Sections 210-20(a), 215-3, and 384-16(d)

Select the proper conductor that complies with Sections 110-14(c), 210-19(a), 215-2, and 230-42(a). Section 110-14(c) requires the circuit conductors to be sized according to Table 310-16. Sections 210-19(a), 215-2 and 230-42(a) required the conductor to be sized no less than 100% of the non-continuous load, plus 125% of the continuous load.

Protect conductors against overcurrent in accordance with Section 240-3. Section 240-3.

Figure 9.00 Conductor and Over Current Protection Tips.

Regardless of the application, conditions and loads must be sized based on the National Electrical Code to avoid damage. A correct protection installation protects and distance from combustible materials all work to minimize the risk of shock, overheating, and fire damage. When you are installing basic electrical components, remember that both your safety and the safety of the people who depend on you are working for are at risk. Since NEC standards are established to ensure installations that are focused on safety compliance is both mandatory and your best way of reducing your professional and personal risk (Figure 9.00).

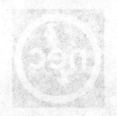

CONDUCTOR AND OVERCURRENT PROTECTION SIZING

Figure 9.00 Conductor and Overcurrent Protection Sizing.

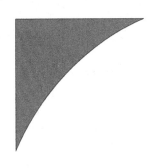

OSHA Regulations Simplified

Failure to comply with the safety standards of the National Electrical Code can result in a failed inspection that can slow the progress of your job. However, if you don't comply with OSHA safety regulations, your entire project can be shut down. Often nonprofit or small, independently owned businesses think they are exempt from OSHA inspections, but they are not. OSHA regulations cover all private-sector employers with one or more workers that engage in any commercial or noncommercial activity that affects commerce. Another misconception by many electrical contractors is that only OSHA 1910, Subpart S applies to them. The truth is that many sections of the OSHA apply to electrical hazards (EHs), including the following:

- 1926.403 Electrical general requirements

- 1926.105 Electrical wiring methods, components, and equipment for general use

- 1910 Subpart I, Personal protective equipment (PPE)

- 1910.137, Electrical protective devices

- 1910.269, Electric power generation, transmission, and distribution

- Shipyard Employment 29 CFR 1915, Subpart L, covering electrical machinery and 1915.181, regarding electrical circuits and distribution boards

- Marine Terminals 29 CFR 1917, Subpart G concerning terminal operations and equipment

OSHA Subpart S for electrical safety falls under the general industry section, rather than the construction industry section of the regulations. The construction industry standards designate the specific conditions required by all construction industry employers. Construction industry employers are legally bound to comply with these standards, as well as any related 29 CFR Part 1910 General Industry standards that also apply. Although 29 CFR 1910 and 1926 are separate standards, some standards are covered in duplicate, and some go into more depth than the other. For example, both 1926 & 1910 cover PPE. While the construction section includes standards on safety belts, lifelines and lanyards, safety nets, and work that takes place on or over water, the general industry standards are more specific about basic PPE such as

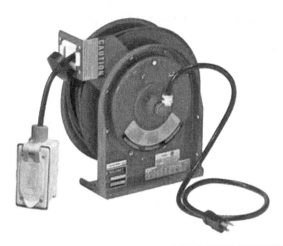

Figure 10.1   Portable ground fault circuit interrupters are a good solution to the GFCI requirement for construction sites.

hardhats and noise protection. OSHA 1926.404(b)(1)(ii) of the construction industry regulations requires the use of ground fault circuit interrupters on all 120-volt outlets used by employees at construction sites that are not part of permanent wiring (Figure 10.1).

GFCIs are not required by the general industry standards. Flame resistant clothing that reflects NFPA 70E requirements is covered in OSHA's General Industry Section 1910.269.

Frequent violation categories

OSHA relies heavily on data and statistics to formulate its regulations and focus its attention on workplace safety. The most frequently violated OSHA construction industry standards include the following categories:

- Aerial lifts (OSHA 1926.453)

- Electrical general requirements (OSHA 1926.403)

- Electrical wiring design and protection (OSHA 1926.404)

- Electrical wiring methods, components, and equipment for general use (OSHA 1926.105)

- Eye and face protection (OSHA 1926.102)

- Fall protection practices (OSHA 1926.502) and fall protection training requirements (OSHA 1926.503)

- General duty requirements (OSHA 5 A 1)

- General safety and health regulations (OSHA 1926.20)

- Head protection (OSHA 1926.100)

- Ladder safety (OSHA 1926.1053)

- Recordkeeping requirements (OSHA 1926.1101)

- Scaffolding safety practices (OSHA 1926.451) and scaffolding training requirements (OSHA 1926.21)

There are many safety compliance issues for the average small company to digest. But OSHA is not some big, bad wolf that lurks in the shadows waiting to pounce on unsuspecting employers. OSHA seeks to identify clear and realistic priorities and to provide employers with the tools and opportunity to protect their workers by emphasizing safety and health. OSHA's purpose is to save lives, prevent workplace injuries and illnesses, and protect the health of all American workers. Whenever possible, OSHA's primary emphasis is on the implementation of hazard control strategies that are based on prevention, and reducing hazardous exposures at their source. For these reasons, OSHA focuses the majority of its field activities on workplaces and job sites where the greatest potential exists for injuries and illnesses.

Specific compliance

Several areas of the OSHA construction industry regulations deal very specifically with electrical installations. OSHA 1926.404 covers wiring methods. A conductor that is used as a grounded conductor must be specifically distinguishable from all other conductors. Grounded conductors cannot be attached to a terminal or lead in a manner that would reverse their designated polarity. Ground-fault circuit interrupters are required on all 120-volt, single-phase 15- and 20-ampere receptacle outlets on construction sites, when the receptacles are not a part of the permanent wiring of the building and could be used by workers. Receptacles on a two-wire, single-phase portable or vehicle-mounted generator not larger than 5 kW (with insulated circuit conductors from the generator frame and all other grounded surfaces) do not have to be protected with ground-fault circuit interrupters. Employers are required to establish and implement an equipment grounding conductor program on construction sites that includes all cord sets, receptacles which are not a part of the building wiring system, and any equipment used by employees that will be connected by cord and plug. All cord sets and cord-and-plug connected equipment must be visually inspected before each day's use for external defects, such as insulation damage, and for possible internal damage. Any damaged or defective equipment must be taken out of service until it is repaired.

OSHA 1926.404(b) (iii) (E) requires equipment to be inspected at the following intervals: before its first use, before being returned to service after any repairs, and every 3 months, except for fixed cord sets and receptacles that are not exposed to damage, which should be inspected every 6 months.

Additionally, a written description of the employer's equipment grounding conductor program and procedures has to be kept on the job site. If a single receptacle is installed on an individual branch circuit it's ampere rating cannot be less than the branch circuit. Unless individual overload protection is used, an attachment plug or receptacle used for cord-and-plug connections of a motor to a branch circuit cannot exceed 15 A at 125 V or 10 A at 250 V.

A disconnect means needs to be provided between all conductors in a building and the service-entrance conductors. Additionally, the disconnecting means must clearly indicate whether it is in the open or closed position and must be installed at a readily accessible location that is close to the service-entrance conductor entry point. Each service disconnecting means also has to be able to simultaneously disconnect all ungrounded conductors. Circuit breakers also need to have a clear indication of whether they are in the open (off) or closed (on) position. Overcurrent devices have to be readily accessible, but they can't be located where they could create an employee safety hazard. An example would be devices that are exposed to physical damage or located in the vicinity of easily ignitable material. If bonding conductors are used to assure electrical continuity, they need to have the capacity to conduct any fault current that might occur.

Power and communication supply lines must be installed with the power lines at the top of the supportive structures and communication lines underneath. This echoes requirements in the NESC. Open conductor clearance requirements in OSHA 1926.404 (C) are as follows:

- 10 feet above finished grade, sidewalks, or from any platform or projection from which they might be reached

- 12 feet over areas subject to vehicular traffic other than truck traffic

- 15 feet over areas other than those subject to truck traffic

- 18 feet over public streets, alleys, roads, and driveways

AC circuits that are less than 50 V that are installed as overhead conductors outside of buildings or supplied by transformers with an ungrounded primary supply system that is less than 150 V to ground must be grounded.

Electric equipment is considered to be effectively grounded per OSHA 1926.404(f)(8)(iii) if it is secured to, and in contact with, a metal rack that provides its support and the metal rack is grounded by the OSHA method specified for the non-current carrying metal parts of fixed equipment.

Personal protective equipment

OSHA requires the use of PPE to reduce employee exposure to hazards. Managing a hazard at its source by using engineered or work practice controls is the best way to protect employees. For example, use of barriers to limit access between an open, energized panel and unqualified personnel is an engineered control. An example of work practice controls would be changing the way employees perform their work, such as wearing PPE. Both employers and employees are responsible for facilitation and use of PPE. Employers are responsible for performing workplace hazard assessments to identify and control physical and health hazards. They must identify the appropriate PPE to be used by employees and train workers in the proper care and use of the PPE. Employees are held responsible for wearing the PPE required for the task at hand, and for its care, cleaning, and maintenance. Additionally, employees have to attend employer PPE training sessions and inform the employer if any PPE needs to be repaired or replaced.

OSHA provides a number of PPE requirements that affect electricians in the field. These include eye and face protection, head protection, foot and leg protection, hand and arm protection, hearing protection, and flame resistant body protection. As the safety officer for one company, I was unpleasantly surprised when visiting job sites to find electricians in sneakers, baseball caps, and with no eye protection in sight. As the benefits administrator for an electrical contracting firm, I would frequently see electricians come in with eye injuries that could have been avoided if they had been wearing eye protection. We even provided our electricians with a choice of safety glasses in a variety of cool styles that included patriotic frames and NFL logos. You are the first line of defense in the field against injuries. As an employer, your company safety manual should include a list of sample tasks and the PPE that you expect workers to wear. Site supervisors are an employer's eyes and voice in the field, and they need to make sure that employees are wearing the required protective equipment. As an employee, all you have to do is wear the appropriate equipment that will protect you from getting hurt. How difficult is it, really, to put on your hardhat and safety glasses before you walk onto a construction site? Let's look at some of the most common types of safety-related PPE that is required by OSHA.

Eye protection

You can't work if you can't see. The majority of eye injuries are the result of not wearing any eye protection or wearing improper or poorly fitted eye guards. Sunglasses, contact lenses, and prescription glasses are not designed to protect your eyes from impacts, dust, insulation fibers, metal fillings, or wires. So don't think that your everyday glasses comply with OSHA safety requirements.

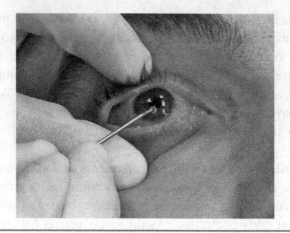

Figure 10.2 Puncture eye injuries can be avoided with proper eye protection.

Eye protection is covered under OSHA 1910.133, which requires employers to ensure that workers use proper eye protection. For example, in work areas where there are potential flying object hazards, the employer must make sure that employees have eye protection with side shields. Flying objects can be as simple as metal filings that pop out from drilling metal studs (Figure 10.2).

Eye injuries are painful just to look at. One accident case I oversaw involved a metal sliver that fell out a beam as an electrician was pulling wire overhead. Puncture wounds can cause severe pain, irritation, infection, and even loss of vision.

There is potential danger from flying objects whenever you are using power tools or performing activities like pushing, pulling, or prying. Additionally, the employer is responsible for ensuring that workers who wear prescription lenses wear eye protection that is designed to take the prescription into consideration. This includes protection such as goggles that can be worn over glasses without disturbing the proper position of the prescription lenses or industrial grade, impact resistant prescription safety glasses. Eye protection should be selected based on potential hazards based on the workplace environment and tasks at hand. They should fit properly and be reasonably comfortable to wear while providing adequate protection (Figure 10.3).

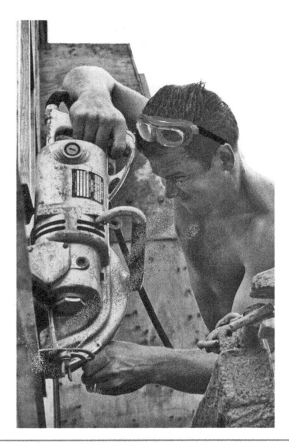

Figure 10.3 If eye protection does not fit properly, workers are not likely to wear it as they should to comply with OSHA requirements.

Head protection

An eye injury can put you out of work for days or weeks, but a head injury can put you out of work permanently, and can even be terminal. Think about this seriously for a minute. Your brain is inside your head and it controls everything your body does. Some worker injuries that have resulted from not wearing a hardhat include permanently blurred vision, memory loss, and lack of coordination. Your neck and spine are connected to your head and an injury to these vital structures can leave you paralyzed for life. OSHA 1910.135 requires that anytime there is the chance of falling overhead objects, tight construction areas where workers could bump their heads on surrounding objects, or the possibility that a worker's head could accidentally come in contact with EHs, an employer must make sure that workers wear head protection. That criteria covers just about any worksite condition.

Hardhats have a hard outer shell and a shock-absorbing lining with a headband and straps that suspend the shell from 1 to 1¼ inches away from your head. The basic design provides ventilation during normal wear and shock absorption in the event of an impact. When you wear a hardhat, the force of a falling object is transmitted and distributed, reducing the impact by approximately 75%. The force of a falling object can be calculated from the weight of the object and the distance that it falls. For example, a metal washer falling about 30 feet will generate a force of 6½ pounds on impact! Now imagine that you are pulling wire in a new construction house and someone working on the trusses two stories above you drops his hammer and it hits your hardhat. This kind of accident has happened more than once, resulting in nothing more than a startled electrician with a few choice words for the carpenter above him. However, without your hardhat to dissipate and absorb that kind of shock, you could end up with a fractured skull or an injury that is so severe it kills you (Figure 10.4).

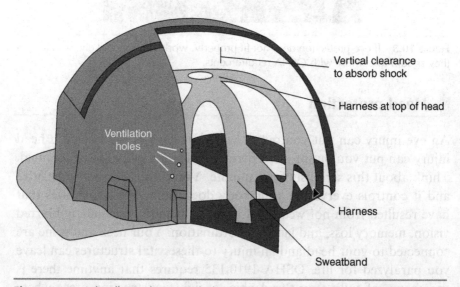

Figure 10.4 A hardhat's design includes a suspension harness that provides impact protection and ventilation.

A true story

Two of our company's electricians went to a job site to install exterior lights on a church while the general contractor was performing repairs on the steeple. They had not started working and were standing on the ground drinking their coffee and chatting with one of the carpenters when a piece of 2 × 4 came falling down from the steeple, bounced off the roof, and headed straight down toward our electricians. George was already wearing his hardhat, but Gary was not. Luckily, the direct impact of the 2 × 4 was absorbed when it hit George's hardhat, but then it ricocheted off of his hardhat and hit Gary. The force of the 2 foot long piece of 2 × 4 startled George but the only harm done was that he spilled his coffee. Unfortunately, Gary ended up with a split in his head that required stitches, as well as a concussion, broken nose, and three shattered teeth. The ER doctor told him that a hardhat would have shielded his face and could have saved him a lot of pain and time lost from work. The moral of the story is that you need to put on your hardhat as soon as you set foot on a construction site. Don't wait until you start working, because other people around you can be the cause of your workplace injury.

Hardhat classifications

Protective headgear must either meet ANSI Standard Z89.1-1986 for protective headgear for industrial workers or provide an equivalent level of protection. Hardhats are divided into three industrial classes as follows:

- *Class A:* These hardhats provide impact and penetration resistance along with limited voltage protection up to 2200 V.

- *Class B:* Hardhats that provide the highest level of protection against EHs, with high-voltage shock and burn protection up to 20,000 V. This classification of helmets also provides protection from impact and penetration hazards from flying or falling objects.

- *Class C:* While these hardhats provide lightweight comfort and impact protection, they do not provide protection from EHs.

Hardhats come in a variety of styles, designs, and colors that can be used by employers to signify employee work classifications. For example, supervisors usually wear white hardhats. If you want your hardhat to make a personal statement, then buy one that comes customized directly from the manufacturer. Never engrave, drill holes into, paint, or apply labels to your hardhat, because it can reduce the integrity of the protection. Excessive exposure to sunlight can also damage your hardhat, so don't store your hardhat in direct sunlight, such as on the rear window shelf of your car. You need to protect the condition of your hardhat so it can properly protect your head. Replace your protective headgear if any of the following types of damage or defects occur:

- Nicks

- Dents

- Gouges

- Cracks

- Fading or obvious dull color

- Loss of surface gloss, chalking, or flaking

- Perforation, cracking, or deformity of the brim or shell

- Exposure to excessive heat, chemicals, or electrical shock (Figure 10.5)

Always replace your hardhat if it sustains an impact, even if there is no visible damage. The outer shell does not have to be cracked or dented to suffer a loss of integrity and protective rating. The majority of manufacturers recommend that you replace your hardhat every 5 years, regardless of whether it has sustained any obvious damage. Manufacture date codes are molded into the hat shell and they specify the day, month, and year that the hardhat was made (Figure 10.6).

The large arrow inside the "month/year" circle points to the month, and the two digits inside that inner circle indicate the year that the hardhat was manufactured. The arrow inside the "day" circle points to the day of the month.

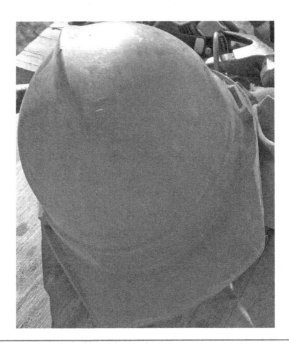

Figure 10.5   Damaged hardhats need to be discarded and replaced.

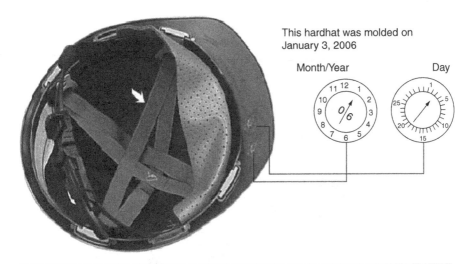

This hardhat was molded on January 3, 2006

Month/Year

Day

Figure 10.6   Hardhat manufacture dates are molded into the brim or inside of the hardhat.

Footwear

If your employees will be working on a site where there is a risk of objects falling, rolling, or piercing the soles of their shoes, then OSHA 1915.156a requires that you make sure workers wear protective footwear. OSHA 1910.136(a) requires protection from these same hazards and adds the risk of employee's feet being exposed to EHs.

OSHA 1915.156(b)(1) stipulates that protective footwear purchased after August 22, 1996 has to comply with ANSI Z41-1991, the American National Standard for Personal Protection-Protective Footwear, or be demonstrated by the employer to be equally as effective as these standards. OSAH 1910.136(b)(1) requires these same compliances, but sets the purchase date for protective footwear that was purchased after July 5, 1994 (Figure 10.7).

OSHA does not consider steel-toe shoes worn by electricians to be hazardous, as long as the conductive portion of the shoe is not in contact with the employee's foot and is not exposed on the outside of the shoe. As an electrician, it is a good idea to consider purchasing non-metallic safety footwear that provides both foot protection and is non-conductive. EH footwear is manufactured with non-conductive electrical shock resistant

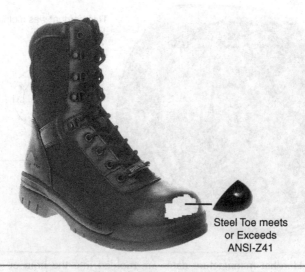

Steel Toe meets
or Exceeds
ANSI-Z41

Figure 10.7 Steel-toe boots provide protection against falling and rolling objects. Non-metallic safety boots are the best choice for electricians.

soles and heals. It is intended to provide a secondary source of protection against accidental contact with live electrical circuits, electrically energized conductors, parts, or apparatus. It must be capable of withstanding the application of 14,000 V at 60 Hz for 1 min with no current flow or leakage current in excess of 3.0 mA, under dry conditions. As an employer, you are not required to pay for ordinary safety-toe footwear so long as you allow employees to wear them off the job site.

Confined space regulations

A confined space has limited or restricted means for entry or exit, and it is not designed for employees to be in continuously. Confined spaces include underground vaults, tanks, storage bins, manholes, and pits. OSHA uses the term "permit-required confined space" or "permit space" to describe a confined space that has the potential to contain a hazardous atmosphere or a material that could engulf an entrant (Figure 10.8).

Additional spaces that would require a permit include those with walls that slope downward and taper into a smaller area that could trap or asphyxiate a worker, or that contain other recognized safety or health hazards, such as unguarded machinery or exposed live wires. OSHA 1910.146 outlines permit-required confined spaces, and Appendix A-F provide such tools as a permit-required confined space decision flow chart and confined space pre-entry checklist (Figure 10.9).

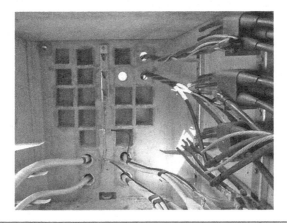

Figure 10.8 Manholes are an example of confined spaces.

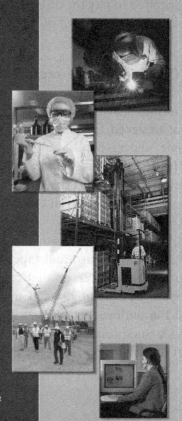

Job Safety and Health
It's the law!

OSHA
Occupational Safety
and Health Administration
U.S. Department of Labor

EMPLOYEES:

- You have the right to notify your employer or OSHA about workplace hazards. You may ask OSHA to keep your name confidential.

- You have the right to request an OSHA inspection if you believe that there are unsafe and unhealthful conditions in your workplace. You or your representative may participate in that inspection.

- You can file a complaint with OSHA within 30 days of retaliation or discrimination by your employer for making safety and health complaints or for exercising your rights under the *OSH Act*.

- You have the right to see OSHA citations issued to your employer. Your employer must post the citations at or near the place of the alleged violations.

- Your employer must correct workplace hazards by the date indicated on the citation and must certify that these hazards have been reduced or eliminated.

- You have the right to copies of your medical records and records of your exposures to toxic and harmful substances or conditions.

- Your employer must post this notice in your workplace.

- You must comply with all occupational safety and health standards issued under the *OSH Act* that apply to your own actions and conduct on the job.

EMPLOYERS:

- You must furnish your employees a place of employment free from recognized hazards.

- You must comply with the occupational safety and health standards issued under the *OSH Act*.

This free poster available from OSHA –
The Best Resource for Safety and Health

Free assistance in identifying and correcting hazards or complying with standards is available to employers, without citation or penalty, through OSHA-supported consultation programs in each state.

1-800-321-OSHA
www.osha.gov

OSHA 3165-12-06R

Figure 10.9 Confined space posters alert workers of the steps involved in confined space entry.

The entry permit that OSHA requires from an employer is a written document that allows and controls entry into a permit space and that contains specific information about the purpose, dates, and duration of entry into the space. The names of authorized entrants, attendants, and the entry supervisor for the permit space must also be listed.

The OSHA entry permit requirement can be met by inserting a reference on the entry permit that notes the means by which authorized workers entering the permit space will be tracked, such as a roster or tracking system.

Your entry permit also needs to list any hazards of the space and the measures you plan to use to isolate the permit space and to eliminate or control hazards before the space is entered. These measures could include lockout or tagging of equipment, ventilating the space, or results of any pre-entry tests that are performed. A list of equipment, such as PPE, testing equipment, communications equipment, alarm systems, and rescue equipment should be provided on the permit as well. Communication procedures that will be used by authorized entrants and attendants to maintain contact during the entry should be outlined on the permit. You also need to have a plan included on the permit for rescue and emergency services, including the equipment to use and the numbers to call for those services.

Before any employees can enter a confined space, OSHA 1910.146(g)(1) requires that they be trained in and possess the understanding, knowledge, and skills necessary for the safe performance of the duties associated with confined space work.

Surviving an OSHA inspection

Even with the best of intentions, circumstances can exist or accidents can happen that result in an OSHA inspection. Keep in mind that OSHA does not just randomly draw company names out of a hat and run out to perform random inspections. OSHA has criteria for determining when an inspection is performed. Obviously, OSHA will respond to fatal or catastrophic workplace injuries, particularly if injuries result in the hospitalization of five or more employees. An inspection will be performed in response to reports of alleged imminent danger situations. OSHA also responds to complaints by employees or union workers or their doctors. But significant media events, such as the rescue of employees from a building collapse, can also prompt an OSHA inspection. Then there are routinely scheduled inspections of high hazard job sites and locations, such as construction of a hospital, or college campus demolitions, renovations and new construction.

Three things typically happen during an OSHA inspection. There is an opening meeting or conference, the actual walk-through inspection, and a closing conference. During the opening meeting, the OSHA Compliance Safety and Health Officer (CSHO) will present his credentials and explain the purpose of the inspection. He may ask to review any job site records such as the OSHA 200 log, or any written programs or safety training records.

All work locations with 11 or more full or part-time employees are required to maintain an OSHA 200 log that records reportable injuries.

THE ROLE OF YOUR SITE REPRESENTATIVE

Regardless of the job site's size, there must be someone present who is an "acting" representative of your company. If you are the owner and you work in the field, who is in charge if you have to leave the job site? The first thing you need to determine when you start a project is the level of supervision required. All of your employees might be perfectly capable of working without a supervisor telling them what to do, but are all of them able to communicate on your company's behalf if an OSHA inspector arrives? Often, large jobs involve a general contractor and a variety of sub-contractors. An OSHA inspector may arrive to review the conditions and receive permission from the general contractor to inspect the site. Since the inspector is already there, he may decide to check out all of the trades onsite. Perhaps OSHA has received a complaint about your work in particular and is only there to inspect you. Either way, you will need to have someone onsite that has been trained in how to facilitate an OSHA inspection, or else you may be opening the door to trouble.

For one thing, the electrical trade involves a number of risks that require a qualified person to be present during work. If you are the qualified person and you leave the site to check on another job, the OSHA inspector will note that there is no trained employee overseeing the work. Another problem is that the average worker often gets very worried when OSHA arrives, and their actions and responses during an inspection can be detrimental and even incriminating. You will want someone representing you who has been trained in the inspection process, and who has access to a camera and a handy-dandy notebook. Let's look at some of your rights and proper actions during an OSHA inspection.

First of all, did you know that OSHA inspectors are empowered to obtain an inspection warrant to gain access to a work site? An inspector is most likely to obtain a warrant before arriving if the examiner believes that a facility will oppose the inspection or if they are responding to a complaint. You have the right to refuse an inspector access to your workplace if he doesn't have a warrant, but the effect is very much like a car salesman refusing to let you test-drive a car before you buy it. At the very least you will probably annoy the inspector and perhaps even raise suspicion that you may have something to hide. Your foreman should be cordial, which is not the same as chummy, and get the inspector's name and office telephone number. Your representative should make a statement to the effect that your company emphasizes safe work practices and then have him ask for, and write down, the reason for the inspection. For example, is it a random visit, a programmed inspection, or in response to a complaint?

If an inspection is related to an employee complaint, your job supervisor should ask for a copy of the complaint. Note that we said ask for a "copy" of the complaint, not just ask for a verbal explanation of the complaint. When you are dealing with OSHA, paperwork is the best way for you to cover your—assets. Although the identity of the person who lodged the complaint may be withheld, you are entitled to know the subject matter of the complaint.

If the visit is not in response to a complaint, your foreman should ask the inspector for a brief explanation of what the inspector plans to inspect and make a note of the explanation. Your representative will also want to ask what workplace records the inspector proposes to review, because an inspector can examine a company's recordkeeping to ensure compliance with OSHA regulations. Here are a number of steps provided by OSHA to their inspectors as guidance for records evaluation:

- Verify the accuracy of the establishment's SIC code and enter the correct SIC code on OSHA 1.

- If you have questions regarding a specific case on the log, request the OSHA 301s or equivalent form for that case.

- Check if the establishment has an onsite medical facility, and where the nearest emergency room is located where employees may be treated.

- Review OSHA Form 300, Log of Work-Related Injuries and Illnesses and assess any repeat instance patterns.

- Ask to see OSHA Form 300 A, Summary of Work-Related Injuries and Illnesses, and review the total hours worked, the number of employees worked for each year, and a roster of current employees.

- Review OSHA Form 301, Injury and Illness Incident Report.

- Verify that the OSHA health and safety poster is posted (Figure 10.10).

Now you know ahead of time what records you need to have on hand.

Following the initial meeting, an OSHA inspector will walk around the job site and take specific note of any complaint hazards or typical compliance issues. Make sure that your job foreman or supervisor takes a camera and goes on the walk-through with the inspector so they have first-hand knowledge of any of the inspector's concerns. If the inspector takes pictures of the site, your foreman needs to take pictures of the same items. If the inspector takes any notes during the site tour, have your representative ask what the inspector has written down and why. Then have your job foreman note the same issues and the inspector's comments. The responsibilities you should expect from your site representative include recording the date and time of the inspection, any documents the inspector reviewed, names of anyone attending the opening and closing conferences, employees who

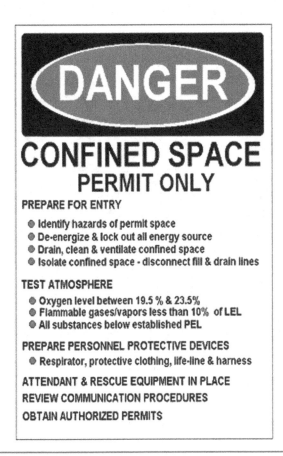

Figure 10.10   The OSHA health and safety poster informs employees of their rights.

were interviewed by the inspector, and areas or equipment that were inspected (Figure 10.11).

All of these proactive steps can help protect you in the event of a citation. Unfortunately, the OSHA inspection is often the time when an employer discovers that they have not been as vigilant or thorough in their risk prevention as they thought or hoped they were. If the inspector finds a problem, make sure your site representative does not admit to any violations, because it could be used against you if you decide to contest the citation.

Common violations that are discovered during a site inspection involve ladders, improper construction of scaffolding, failure to provide adequate fall protection for employees working at heights, and the absence

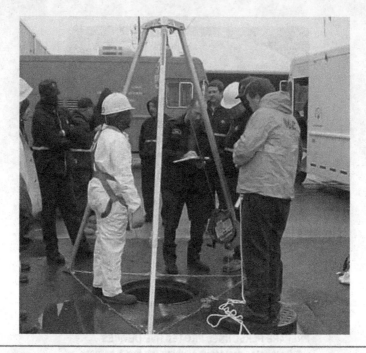

Figure 10.11 Your job supervisor is your representative during an OSHA inspection and should take notes about the inspection.

of guards around workplace hazards. Typical violations that are specifically related to the electrical trade are improper use of flexible extension cords or using damaged, cut, or taped extension cords, inadequate lockout/tagout methods, unguarded energized conductors, absence of ground fault protection on construction sites, and failure to use proper PPE (such as hardhats, gloves, or flash suits). Improper installation of lights or electrical equipment that is used to provide electric power at the job site is also a common violation. The OSHA inspector will often allow you the opportunity to rectify these issues and schedule a follow-up walk-through to ensure that problem areas have been addressed.

THE NIGHTMARE OF AN OSHA VIOLATION

If your company is cited by OSHA for a standard violation, you may be assessed a fine. This is not like getting a $10 parking ticket. For example, in June 2008, OSHA cited a commercial contracting company for fall hazards at a 77 Unit condominium construction project and proposed $877,000 in penalties. There are several types of OSHA citations. A willful citation is issued for violations committed with disregard or indifference to the Occupational Safety and Health Act and regulations. A violation under Section 17(a) of the OSH Act will result in a repeat violation. OSHA issues a repeat violation when it finds a substantially similar violation of any standard, rule, or order that was previously cited at any of an employer's facilities. A repeat violation can carry with it a fine of up to $70,000 per violation, per employer facility. As you can see, prevention and compliance are well worth your time, effort, and enforcement. Complaining or even proving that an OSHA standard was burdensome will not get you out of a citation. To prove the validity of a citation, OSHA only needs to prove the following:

- That the employer violated the general duty clause or any other OSHA standard

- That employees were exposed to the offending condition

- That the employer had actual or constructive knowledge of the offending condition

The fact that employees had access to the offending condition and that the employer had knowledge of the condition are both relatively easy for OSHA to prove. All OSHA has to do is note that a normally diligent employer should have known about the citation condition, and then it immediately follows that is was "reasonably predictable" that an employee would be exposed to the violating condition, even if just accidentally. OSHA violations can result in fines of up to $7000 per day for each hazard that is not resolved, and willful or repeated violations can have fines of up $70,000 per violation. If OSHA cites an employer for a willful violation, it must prove that the employer acted with reckless disregard for OSHA requirements.

There are a few ways that you can defeat an OSHA citation. For example, if you could prove that complying with an OSHA standard was impossible, or that compliance would have posed a greater hazard to employees than noncompliance, you might be able to overturn a citation. This type of affirmative defense requires proof that no other alternate means of protection was viable and that is a point that is extremely difficult to make.

Even willful employee negligence or misconduct is difficult to prove, because, as a general rule, OSHA considers employers responsible for the actions of their employees. In order to have a chance at getting a citation repealed that was caused by an employee's unsafe actions, you would have to prove that you had adopted and trained the worker in safety means that would prevent an OSHA violation. Additionally, you would need to show that, as a safety conscious employer, you regularly and diligently sought to discover and rectify any instances of non-compliance and that you implement actions to deter violations, such as suspension or termination of anyone violating your company's safety rules. Telling OSHA that you had verbally reprimanded the offending employee in the past will not meet the burden of proof. Immediately you can see why a thorough and effective safety policy and documented training is so important to you as an employer. If your job supervisor sees any employees violating even the most basic safety requirements, such as not wearing a hardhat, he needs to follow your safety plan rules to the letter. Looking the other way, or making allowances "just this once" for an employee's risky behavior will make it impossible for you to use a willful misconduct defense.

Contesting an OSHA Citation

As a rule of thumb, it is advisable to contest an OSHA violation. You may be thinking that it would be better not to make waves with OSHA, but the reality is that the worst thing that can happen during an OSHA hearing is that you lose the case and still have to pay the same fines that would have been assessed if you had not tried to contest the violation. Here are a couple of facts to consider. An OSHA inspector has no way of knowing whether you are a conscientious employer who emphasizes safe work practices, or some fly-by-night company that just wants to get their money fast and the heck with site risks or hazards. Any employer can profess to an OSHA inspector that safety is a priority to them, but the proof is in the documentation. Another reason to consider contesting a citation is to avoid a repeat violation citation and the increased fines associated with that level of infraction. Third-party lawsuits are another risky result of an OSHA citation. Some states, such as Massachusetts, grant employees double compensation if their injuries are the result of "serious and willful misconduct." In this example, it is the employer, not his or her insurance carrier, who must pay the extra compensation. During a violation hearing, the OSHA representative's role is to demonstrate that the employer was negligent and, in other words "willfully," non-compliant.

OSHA's area directors are authorized to enter into settlement negotiations that revise citations and penalties. This level of negotiations must take place and be concluded within 15 working days of the employer's receipt of the citations. You have to present compelling evidence that convinces the area director, the inspector, and possibly the inspector's supervisor that the facts supposedly observed at the work place are not accurate.

It may be possible for you to negotiate a 15% penalty reduction if you agree to develop and implement a safety and health management program. OSHA may reduce penalties for an employer who currently has a safety and health management program in place. If, during the course of the hearing, your program is deemed to be defective, a 25% penalty reduction can still be granted, and even ineffective programs may quality for a 15% penalty reduction. Another means of reducing a proposed penalty is to provide proof that the business is unable to pay the full amount, even if payments are spread over time. OSHA's area director has discretion to determine when a penalty should be reduced based upon an employer's financial condition. OSHA penalties are designed to provide a deterrent effect, not to punish employers or raise revenue for the government.

SURVIVING AN OSHA HEARING

If you decide to contest a violation and go before the administrative law judge, you have the opportunity to present your safety policy, training records, and even personnel attendance and your workers' compensation MOD report as proof that you strive to be a diligent, safe employer. To fight a citation, you must file a written contest within 15 calendar days of receipt of the OSHA notice of the proposed penalty. Your response needs to include that you are challenging either the violation or proposed penalty, or both. Even if you choose to contest a violation, you are still required to post the citation at or near the work area involved. The citation must remain posted until the violation has been corrected or for three working days, whichever is longer.

OSHA has the burden of convincing the judge that it has the "greater weight of evidence" and to prove all of the elements of a citation. Don't get too excited about this preponderance of evidence because all OSHA has to establish to win the case is that you should have known about a violation. So why would you go to the trouble of contesting a violation? Because you can argue to have the citation repealed completely, have the amount of the penalty reduced, or extend the abatement period. If you file a notice to contest, it delays the running of the abatement period, so if nothing else it buys you time to fix the violation.

When you arrive at your hearing, be sure to bring any test results you have conducted, a copy of your safety manual, training records, field notes, written personnel statements from site workers, and any pictures that your foreman took when the OSHA inspector did his walk-through of the job site. Now it is time for you to show the judge that you are a proactive, safety conscious employer. First, demonstrate your commitment to safety and to employee involvement and compliance. Summarize your safety policies, including safety meetings and routine OSHA compliant training. Provide records that your company performs hazard analysis and implements risk controls. Basically, you are making the case that the conditions that caused a violation were extremely unusual based on your company's commitment to safe work practices.

Even if you come off smelling like a rose, you may not succeed in having the citation repealed, but you may be able to negotiate a lower penalty. Obviously, the best way to ensure that you do not receive a citation or penalty is to avoid violations through safety compliance. Keep your job sites free of hazards, make sure that all employees understand their obligation to wear appropriate PPE, provide regular trainings and safety meetings, only allow qualified workers to perform restricted tasks, and know your responsibilities under the key OSHA standards that apply to electrical work and general duty (Figure 10.00).

OSHA RESOURCES

Occupational Safety & Health Administration
200 Constitution Avenue, NW
Washington, DC 20210

 Compliance Assistance Specialists

 Laws & Regulations

 Synopsis of the OSH Act

 OSHA Cooperative Programs

 Frequently Asked Questions

Compliance Assistance Resources

- o eTools
- o Safety and Health Topics Pages
- o Brochures and Booklets
- o Fact Sheets
- o Posters
- o Safety and Health Information Bulletins (SHIBs)
- o Technical Manual
- o Training and Reference Materials Library
- o Training Videos

- o NIOSH Health Hazard Evaluation Program
- o On-site Consultation Program
- o Sample Programs

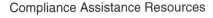

Figure 10.00 OSHA Resources On-line and in Print.

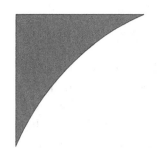

Chapter 11

Accident and Injury Prevention and Procedures

Chapter Outline

251

The most beneficial and money-saving partnership for a construction business is when both the employer and employees work together to make safety the company's top priority. Lots of organizations and workers pay this practice lip service, but they do not really believe that safety should come before deadlines, bonuses, production, or profits. All of that changes when a worker gets hurt and groups such as workers' compensation, OSHA, distraught family members, doctors, and lawyers get involved.

Sometimes it is the simplest of precautions that can return the greatest results. Often employees will be mindful of major safety practices such as energized work procedures, arc blast protection, and installing conduit in trenches, but they won't take the time to focus on repetitious movements, ear protection, ladder safety, or basic first aid.

Ergonomics, not just for office workers

Mention the term "ergonomics" and most electricians think about the company secretaries who spend their day performing data entry for hours at a time. Ergonomics is a human engineering discipline that addresses the effect that work environments and tasks have on employees. The idea behind ergonomics is to understand pressure and stress that is exerted on different parts of the body as a consequence of specific tasks, and to identify, prevent or alleviate injuries that can result from these actions.

Musculoskeletal disorders (MSDs), including carpal tunnel syndrome (CTS), are an example of work-related ergonomic injuries that account for 14% of doctor's visits and 19% of hospital stays nationwide. Of the people who develop MSDs, 62% report some degree of activity limitation. Repetitive stress injury (RSI) is a comprehensive term for a variety of disorders that cause damage to tendons, nerves, bones, and muscles due to the repeated performance of a limited number of physical movements. Some of the symptoms of RSI are numbness, tingling, pain, swelling, burning, loss of dexterity, and muscle weakness. Other terms associated with RSI include: Cumulative Trauma Disorder (CTD), Occupational Overuse Syndrome (OOS), Repetitive Motion Syndrome

(RMS), CTS, and Tendonitis. Repetitive stress injuries cost employers over $80 billion a year. Just the average compensation of an employee suffering from CTS is $33,000.00.

One of the most common parts of the body that is affected by RSI is the hand. When you tense a muscle to just 50% of its ability, the blood flowing through the capillaries in the muscle can be completely shut off. Repeated tensing of your hand can cause the fibers of the tendons running through the carpal tunnel to separate or break. This causes friction between the tendon and its sheath and ultimately results in tendonitis. Typical early symptoms include numbness, or tingling or burning sensations in the fingers, hands, forearms, elbows, and even the shoulder and neck. Ask anyone who put off having carpal tunnel surgery and they will tell you that this condition can become crippling. Victims of full-blown RSI have reported that they cannot wash their own hair or even hold a sheet of paper without agonizing pain. One of the problems with diagnosing these conditions in tradesmen is that electricians and other construction workers expect to have some degree of pain at the end of a hard day's work, and so they don't or won't recognize the early warning signs of RSI (Figure 11.1).

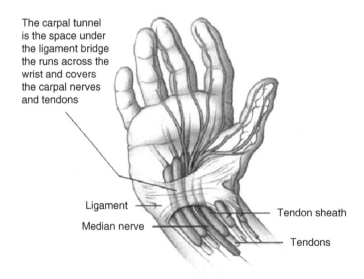

The carpal tunnel is the space under the ligament bridge the runs across the wrist and covers the carpal nerves and tendons

Ligament

Median nerve

Tendon sheath

Tendons

Figure 11.1 Carpal tunnel syndrome is a painful condition that can restrict your ability to grasp or use tools.

As an electrician, if you are still not convinced that any of this pertains to you, then maybe we should look at some of the causes of repetitive stress injuries. These include:

- Overuse of the muscles on a continued repetitive basis
- Cold temperatures
- Vibrating equipment
- Forceful activities
- Poor posture, awkward body positioning, kneeling for long periods of time
- Holding the same posture on a continuous basis
- Prolonged periods of work without a break
- Direct pressure or a blow to the body
- Carrying heavy loads on a repeated basis
- Fatigue

Do any of those characteristics describe aspects of your job? Tendonitis often develops amongst electricians because of the repetitive wrist extension, flexing, and thrust necessary to grip wire strippers, screwdrivers, and other hand tools (Figure 11.2).

Installing and maintaining temporary wiring systems on construction sites often requires a worker to work with their hands at or above shoulder height. Overhead work can cause MSDs such as tendonitits of the shoulder, and lifting can cause MSDs of the back and shoulders. The worker may also experience neck pain or injury because the neck is frequently in an extreme position during overhead work to allow the worker to see what he is doing (Figure 11.3).

MSDs are the most common injuries in the construction industry, accounting for over one-third of all lost workday injuries and about half of all compensation claims. Electricians who install and maintain temporary wiring systems can develop rotator cuff tendonitis, low back pain from lifting materials overhead, and tension neck syndrome.

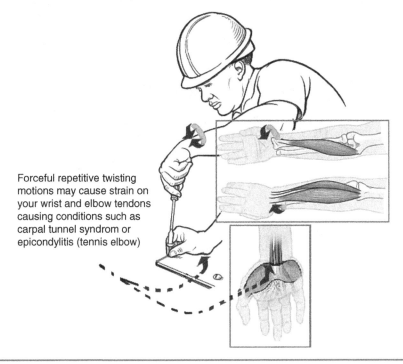

Forceful repetitive twisting motions may cause strain on your wrist and elbow tendons causing conditions such as carpal tunnel syndrom or epicondylitis (tennis elbow)

Figure 11.2 Using a screwdriver for just an hour can result in a repetitive stress injury.

Tension neck syndrome is characterized by pain in the shoulder and neck region, accompanied by tenderness over the shoulder-neck muscles. It is one of the most common work-related MSDs of the neck and shoulder.

Ergonomic assessment and injury prevention

An effective safety program will identify potential work injuries and provide alternative work methods to avoid them. For example, heavy loads such as large spools of wire bundles of conduit, or heavy tools and machinery place great stress on muscles, discs, and vertebrae. Lifting any load that is heavier than about 50 pounds will increase the risk of injury, particularly if you lift and twist or if proper lifting postures are not used. Everyone should be trained in the right way to lift a load, and to use forklifts or duct lifts to lift articles such as heavy spools, transformers, switch gears, service sections,

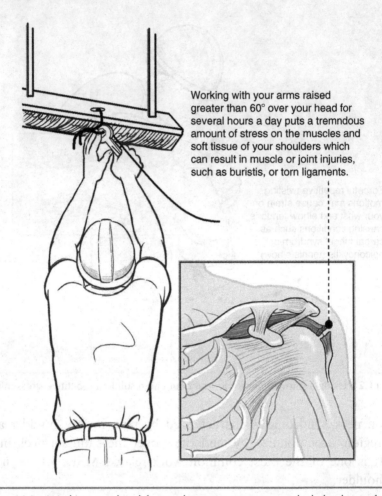

Working with your arms raised greater than 60° over your head for several hours a day puts a tremndous amount of stress on the muscles and soft tissue of your shoulders which can result in muscle or joint injuries, such as buristis, or torn ligaments.

Figure 11.3 Working overhead for too long can cause musculoskeletal or soft tissue injuries.

conduit, and machinery. Opt to use ramps or lift gates to load machinery into trucks instead of lifting it up and into the vehicle (Figure 11.4).

Bending while lifting forces your back to support the weight of your upper body in addition to the weight you are lifting. Bending over at the waist while you are lifting an object, even something as light as a screwdriver, places excessive strain on you back. Carrying loads on one shoulder, under one arm, or in one hand, creates uneven pressure on the spine. There are some simple solutions to these situations. For

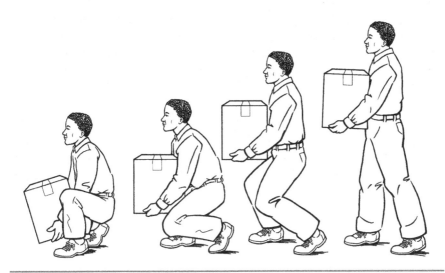

Figure 11.4   If you have to lift a load, do so by bending at the knees, not the waist, and keep your spine in a neutral, straight spine alignment whenever possible. Materials that must be manually lifted should be placed at "power zone" height, which is about mid-thigh to mid-chest.

example, move as close to the object as possible, and use your legs when lifting. Also, keep your elbows close to your body and keep the load as close to your body as possible.

At some point during any electrical work you are likely to have to work over your head to pull wire, install a junction box, or hang a fixture. Holding even light items over your head for a long period of time increases the risk of back and shoulder injury, because muscles become starved of nutrients, blood flow is reduced, and waste products can build up in your bloodstream. One easy and inexpensive way to eliminate activities such as holding a piece of equipment overhead while you are drilling mounting holes is to make a template out of cardboard first and drill the holes from that. Another way of reduced prolonged overhead work is to rotate employees every hour so that no one person is exposed to the same activity for too long. Work in teams and have one person hold an item while the other person installs it. This will decrease the amount of time it takes for the installation and reduce the risk of injuries such as falling, flying objects, drilling incidents, and overall stress on the body.

Take regular breaks and break tasks into shorter segments. This will give muscles adequate time to rest. Working through breaks increases the risk of MSDs, accidents, and reduces the quality of work because employees are over-fatigued.

All electricians have to pull some kind of wire. Larger gauge wire requires a greater exertion to pull due to its increased weight and stiffness. This effort causes stress on your hands, arms, shoulders, and back and increases the risk of puncture injuries and falls. Pulling wire through bends in conduit causes points of restriction which increase the amount of force required to perform the task.

A good alternative is to use a mechanical wire-puller which can provide the force of several workers, increasing productivity and reducing the risk of muscles pulls. If you have to pull cable manually, take regular breaks to allow your muscles to rest and be sure to wear gloves to improve your grip and protect your hands from cuts and friction. Lubricating wires that go through chases, conduits, or knockouts will also reduce friction and decrease the pulling force required.

Ergonomics and hand tools

Poorly designed hand tools force you to use awkward grip postures that can result in tendonitis in your hands, wrists, and elbows. Even something as simple as short handles on hand tools can press or rub against your palm and fingers causing contact stress to the inside and outside of your hand. Tools with wide handle spans force you to extend thumb and finger positions to activate the tool, which also stresses your hand, wrist, and forearms (Figure 11.5).

If you don't position tools like drills directly in front of your mid-section, the drill can slip and injure you or put unnecessary pressure on your back. Generally, an inline tool is best on horizontal surfaces at about waist height, and a pistol grip is preferable for vertical surfaces at about waist height. Even using a screwdriver for a long period of time can cause damage to your joints and tendons. Choose

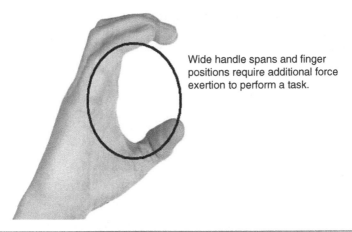

Wide handle spans and finger positions require additional force exertion to perform a task.

Figure 11.5 If your hand makes the letter "C" when you grasp a drill or other hand tool, you are putting exertion on your hand that can cause tendon injuries.

screwdrivers that have handles that are between 1 1/2 to 3 inches in diameter, with triangular handles with rounded edges to provide a better grip. You can reduce hand strain by using tools with padded grips and handles that extend across the whole palm of the hand to minimize contact pressure. Minimize the period of time you continuously use a vibrating tool to 10-15 minutes and no more than 2 hours of total operation time per day.

Stretches

Anyone can stop and do simple ergonomic stretches for a few minutes every couple of hours. Stretching is designed to eliminate pressure points on your wrists, shoulders, hands, neck, and back and reduce your risk of repetitive movement or excessive stress strain. You don't have to look like you are doing yoga or use your entire break in order to effectively stretch. Simply tipping your head forward and back several times, slowly shrugging your shoulders five times or reaching behind your head and gently tugging on your elbow are simple, beneficial ways of stretching (Figures 11.6 and 11.7).

BACK TO FRONT HEAD NECK STRETCHES

1. Tip your head back slowly

2. Hold for 5 seconds

3. Slowly tip head forward

4. Hold for 5 seconds

5. Repeat 5 times

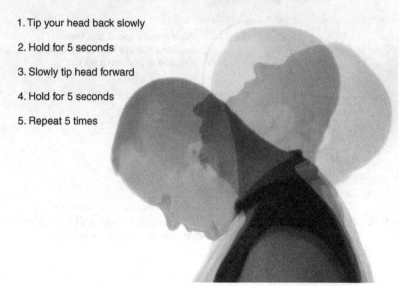

Figure 11.6   Relax the pressure on your shoulders and neck with head tips.

ELBOW PRESS

1. Put your right hand over and behind your left shoulder. Press gently on your right elbow with your left hand. Hold for 20 seconds.

2. Relax your arms for 5 seconds.

3. Put your left hand over and behind your right shoulder. Press gently on your left elbow with your right hand. Hold for 20 seconds.

4. Relax your arms.

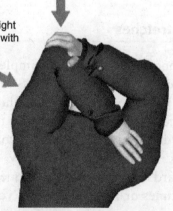

Figure 11.7   Relax stress on your arms, shoulders, and back with elbow pulls.

Safety DOs and DON'Ts

I wish I could tell you that workers have an intuitive safety sense when it comes to the basics, such as ladder use, hard hats, ear protection, and drilling, but all too often people let deadlines or budgets distract them from essential safety practices. Imagine that you have only scheduled a few days to rough-in a new house, but the carpenters are running behind schedule and then your materials are delivered late. If you were behind the eight ball and strapped for time, would you still take the time to be safety conscious? This is the real life challenge. On paper, a safety policy is a great idea, but it is only a beneficial tool if you use it.

So instead of talking in theory, let's look at some practical ways for you to fit safety into your busy day. A must for every one of your job sites and each company truck is an emergency checklist. This form should include the name and address of the current job site and the nearest hospital. All too often people call 911 for help and can't tell them the address where they are working. Blurting out that you are working at the University of Maine in Augusta and then trying to give directions while you are also trying to assess someone's injury or offer assistance will only impede the response time of professional help. The checklist should also include simple instructions, like contacting the job foreman so he or she can gather up the injured employee's personal belongings, and reporting the incident to the office so they can contact the person's family and file any necessary claims with the insurance company. If it is your company's policy that a worker who has been in a vehicular accident contacts the police or auto insurer, then list that as well. Time is of the essence when it comes to certain procedures following an accident of any kind, and a checklist will help to make sure all the bases are covered without creating additional down time.

We already discussed that eye protection and hard hats are required personal protection, but here are a couple of tips to get you to use them everyday. Strap your hard hat to your tool belt or box at the end of every workday so it will be ready for you to put on each morning when you grab your tools. Keep a supply of lanyard style

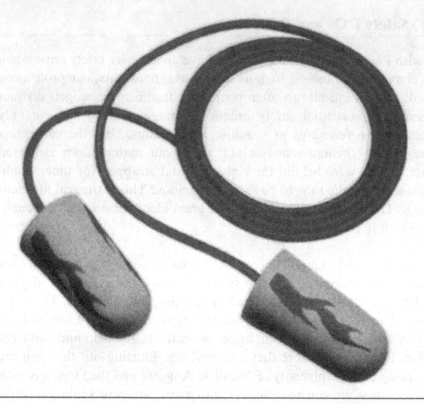

Figure 11.8 OSHA approved earplugs come in a variety of different styles, colors, and patterns.

or U-band earplugs on your dresser and toss them around your neck when you get dressed everyday. You can even get them in a variety of colors or patterns, like flames, so they have a little style. Hey, it's better than wearing a tie, and after a few times, putting in your earplugs will become as automatic as putting on your shirt (Figure 11.8).

Or you can toss a set of wrapped earplugs inside your gloves so that when you put your work gloves on you have to take the earplugs out, which will remind you to put them in. One more important point— Your earplugs can't protect your ears if you don't put them in properly. It is as easy as roll, pull, and hold. Hold the earplug between your thumb and forefinger and start to roll and compress the entire earplug to a small, crease-free cylinder. While you are rolling the earplug, take your other hand and reach over your head and pull up and back on your outer ear. This will straighten out your ear canal so the earplug will fit snuggly.

> If you always seem to have problems getting plugs into your ear so they fit properly, try opening your mouth while you put them in. Some people need this extra step to straighten out their ear cannel enough for the plug to go in straight and expand fully.

Insert the earplug and hold it in place with the end of your finger while you count to 30 to give the ear plug enough time to expand and fill your ear canal. When you are finished wearing them, remove your earplugs slowly, twisting them in one direction to break the seal. If you remove your earplugs too quickly or just yank them out, you can create a vacuum and damage your eardrum (Figure 11.9).

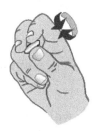

1. Roll   the earplug up into a small, thin "snake" with your fingers. You can use one or both hands.

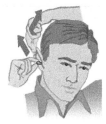

2. Pull   the top of your ear up and back with your opposite hand to straighten out your ear canal. The rolled-up earplug should slide right in.

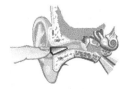

3. Hold   the earplug in with your finger. Count to 20 or 30 out loud while waiting for the plug to expand and fill the ear canal. Your voice will sound muffled when the plug has made a good seal.

Figure 11.9   Use caution to properly insert earplugs.

Now to protect your eyes. Many of our electricians chose to buy neck straps for their safety glasses so they were always accessible. When you lean over to pick up the first tool, your glasses will be hanging right there in front of you and it will be easier and less cumbersome to put them on than to leave them tangling off your neck. If you will be wearing a safety shield, put it in the same bag with your flame retardant cover shirt or attach it to your insulated hand tool bag. That way you can't use one form of protection without the other.

Ladders

A ladder is one of the easiest tools you will use in the construction industry, but accidents involving ladders send more than 222,000 people to emergency rooms each year. So how is it that something so simple ends up being so dangerous? Most ladder accidents are caused by negligence or failure to use the proper ladder for the task at hand. OSHA takes ladder safety so seriously that under OSHA 29 CFR 1926, Sub Part X, employers are required to provide a training program for any employees who will be using ladders.

Use fiberglass ladders whenever there is a possibility of working near electricity or overhead power lines.

One of the first steps in ladder safety is to use a ladder with the proper duty rating to carry the combined weight of the worker and any material being installed.

Following are the four categories of ladder duty ratings.

Type I These ladders have a duty rating of 250 pounds. Type I ladders are manufactured for heavy-duty use.

Type IA These ladders have a duty rating of 300 pounds. Type IA ladders are recommended for extra-heavy-duty industrial use.

Type II These ladders have a duty rating of 225 pounds. Type II ladders are approved for medium-duty use.

Type III These ladders have a duty rating of 200 pounds. Type III ladders are rated for light-duty use.

Type IA and Type I ladders are the only acceptable ladders on a construction job site.

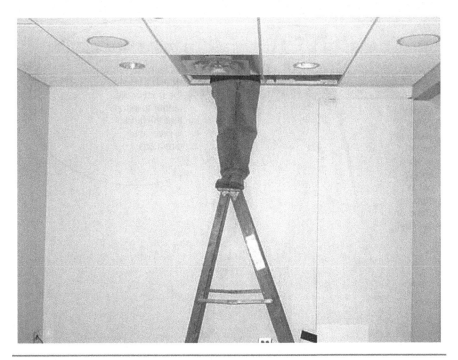

Figure 11.10 Never stand on the top platform of a stepladder. The odds of falling are dramatically increased.

Be sure to use the proper size ladder for the job at hand (Figure 11.10).

The average electrician will usually be most comfortable working at his shoulder level, which is about 5 feet above where he stands. Since you are required to stand at least 2 feet down from the top of a ladder to be safe, the maximum working height would be about 3 feet above the top of the ladder (5 feet minus 2 feet). For example, a 5-foot stepladder would give an effective working height of 8 feet (5 feet plus 3 feet). If you will be working off a straight or extension ladder, you need to stand 3 feet down from the top, which gives an effective working height of 2 feet above the ladder top.

For every 4 feet of extension ladder height, the bottom of the ladder should be 1 foot away from the wall or object it is leaning against. Be sure that metal steps and rungs are grooved or roughened to prevent slipping. On a stepladder, ensure that the spreaders, the devices that hold the front and back sections in an open position, are completely open and locked

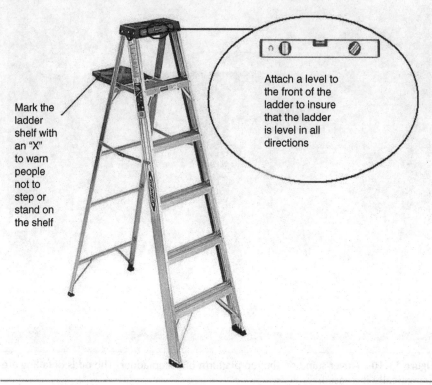

Mark the ladder shelf with an "X" to warn people not to step or stand on the shelf

Attach a level to the front of the ladder to insure that the ladder is level in all directions

Figure 11.11   Stepladder safety is something you can encourage.

before putting any weight on the ladder. One trick of the trade I have seen electricians use to encourage ladder safety is to remove or mark the tool shelf on a stepladder to eliminate the risk that someone will stand on it. Another electrician I know attached a level to his stepladder so that he knows it will not wobble or tip while he is working from it (Figure 11.11).

First aid

Simple first aid can reduce the physical damage caused by an accident or even save a life. The first reaction you need to have if you or someone else gets injured is to stay calm and use your head. You cannot render aid if you don't stop and take the time to follow a few basic safety steps. This is particularly true if someone has received an electrical shock from a live wire. Running in and grabbing a person who is in contact with electrical current will only put you in danger as well. You can also cause additional damage to an injured person by not thinking your way through assisting them. Moving someone with a back or neck injury, for example, can paralyze them. Driving someone who has just cut off a finger to the emergency room without also bringing the amputated finger means you have eliminated that person's chance of having re-attachment surgery.

Do not place a severed finger or other body part directly in a bag of ice or cooler filled with ice. This can freeze and damage the tissue. Instead, wrap the finger in a *clean*, moistened cloth, put that in a bag, and then put the bag in ice. This creates a barrier to direct contact with the freezing ice, while keeping the finger cool. Generally, human tissues will survive for about 6 hours without any cooling, and approximately 12 hours if cooled.

Everyone can benefit from basic first aid knowledge, but for people who work in a trade that is filled with risks and hazards, first aid is a safety necessity. The main thing to remember with first aid is—first things first. When someone gets hurt you need to quickly assess the situation, call for help, and then render any assistance that you can without putting yourself in harm's way. You will need to remember to tell emergency responders what happened to the victim, symptoms or injuries that you observed, and any steps you took to provide first aid. Some injuries are easier to treat than others, so let's start by looking at some of these.

Bleeding

Bleeding needs to be stopped quickly before the injured person goes into shock or loses a critical amount of blood. First, grab a clean cloth, put it over the person's wound and apply direct pressure. Elevate the area of the body that is bleeding. For example, if someone cuts his/her arm, apply pressure and hold the arm up in the air. Gravity, combined with pressure, will help reduce the blood flow until medical assistance arrives. Avoid applying a tourniquet, because if you make it too tight you can cut off the blood flow to the arm completely.

Carry a zip-lock baggy with a clean cloth or sanitary wipes in your lunchbox or toolbox in case someone gets cut or burned. Keeping injuries clean on a construction site is key to preventing infection.

Eye injury

Eye injuries are painful for the victim, and often their first reaction is to rub the affected eye. This is the worst thing they could do. If dust, dirt, or chemicals have gotten into a person's eye, the first treatment should be to immediately flush the eye with water for at least 5 minutes. If you are nowhere near an eye wash station, have the person hold open the eye and tip the head sideways and gently pour water on the corner of the eye. Do not use medications advertised to clear red eyes. After rinsing the eye, cover both eyes with a clean cloth and seek immediate medical assistance, even if the person says they feel fine. Grit can scratch the eye's surface, which may require antibiotic treatment, and chemicals will burn the eye's surface.

If something gets stuck in a person's eye do not attempt to rinse the eye. Instead, cover the injured eye with paper, plastic, or a styrofoam cup, and cover the other eye with a clean cloth. Why do you need to cover the uninjured eye? Because our eyes blink in tandem, and this will keep them from blinking and causing additional damage to the punctured eye (Figure 11.12).

Electrical shock

Earlier in this book we looked at the hazards posed by electrical current, and the dangers involved with coming in contact with live conductors. Many electricians have received a jolt when they inadvertently came in contact with an energized part. Even non-trades people have been shocked when they touched a lamp with loose wiring or plugged in an appliance that was already turned on.

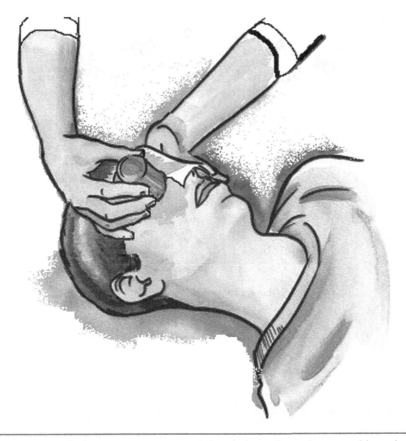

Figure 11.12 Placing a cup over an eye injury helps to keep the eye stable and prevent the victim from disturbing the eye.

It leaves people thinking that it must take a tremendous level of current to really hurt someone, but this is far from true. It only takes half an ampere of direct contact with electricity to cause cardiac arrest (Figure 11.13).

As long as a person is in contact with live current you cannot safely administer any form of first aid without risking your own safety. It is easy to panic when you see someone being electrocuted, but it is critical that you use your head and stay calm. First, disconnect the power source if you can do so safely and call for help. If you cannot turn off the power, find an insulated material like a phone book, piece of plywood, or insulating mat to stand on

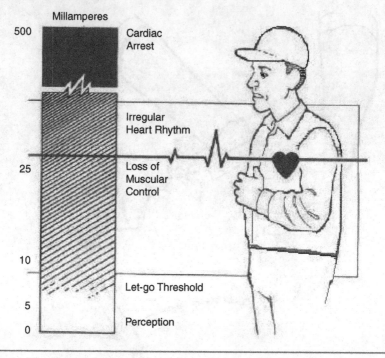

Figure 11.13 Shock levels cause loss of muscle control and heart attack.

and then use a piece of wood, wooden broom handle, dry rope, or a hot stick to break the connection between the victim and the power source (Figure 11.14).

Do not try to move a victim who is in contact with a high voltage wire, such as a downed power line, even if you have access to high-voltage gloves. If any unprotected part of your body comes in contact with the high voltage current, you will become a victim too. Unless you know the voltage, which is usually a minimum of 45 kV for high power conductors, you have no way of knowing if even a hot stick is safe to use. Most hot sticks that electricians have on their trucks are rated at only 2, 6, or 11 kV.

Many victims of electrocution will receive burns, go into shock, or suffer a heart attack.

Treat burned areas by covering them with a clean, damp cloth until help arrives. Signs that someone is going into shock include agitation,

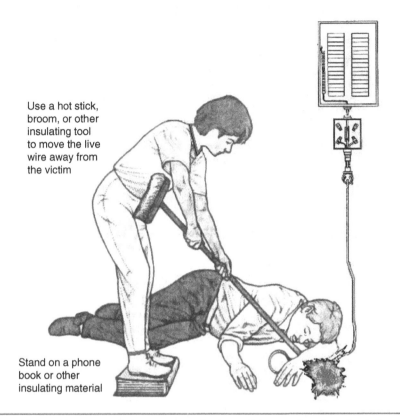

Use a hot stick, broom, or other insulating tool to move the live wire away from the victim

Stand on a phone book or other insulating material

Figure 11.14 You cannot help someone who is receiving an electrical shock if you do not take precautions to ensure your own safety as well.

confusion and disorientation, dizziness, difficultly remaining conscious, and shallow breathing. You would probably expect anyone who was just electrocuted to be jittery and disoriented. Rather than try to determine if the victim is going into shock, treat him/her as if they are in shock. Lay the person on his/her back and elevate the legs about 12 inches off the floor. Do not put a pillow or folded shirt under the head, because you do not want to elevate the head. Cover the injured person with a blanket or jackets to maintain warmth and loosen any tight clothing around the neck, wrists, and waist. If the person begins to vomit or drool, turn his/her head to one side to avoid choking. If the victim's lips turn blue, they stop breathing, or they show symptoms of a heart attack, follow the first aid steps for a heart attack (Figure 11.15).

Electrical Shock - First Aid Steps

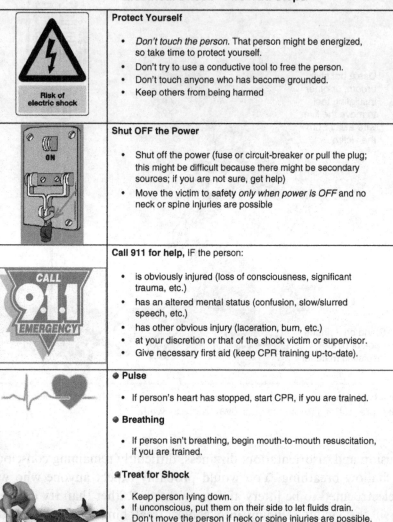

	Protect Yourself • _Don't touch the person._ That person might be energized, so take time to protect yourself. • Don't try to use a conductive tool to free the person. • Don't touch anyone who has become grounded. • Keep others from being harmed
	Shut OFF the Power • Shut off the power (fuse or circuit-breaker or pull the plug; this might be difficult because there might be secondary sources; if you are not sure, get help) • Move the victim to safety _only when power is OFF_ and no neck or spine injuries are possible
	Call 911 for help, IF the person: • is obviously injured (loss of consciousness, significant trauma, etc.) • has an altered mental status (confusion, slow/slurred speech, etc.) • has other obvious injury (laceration, burn, etc.) • at your discretion or that of the shock victim or supervisor. • Give necessary first aid (keep CPR training up-to-date).
	Pulse • If person's heart has stopped, start CPR, if you are trained. **Breathing** • If person isn't breathing, begin mouth-to-mouth resuscitation, if you are trained. **Treat for Shock** • Keep person lying down. • If unconscious, put them on their side to let fluids drain. • Don't move the person if neck or spine injuries are possible. • Cover the person to maintain body heat and elevate legs 12 inches

Figure 11.15 Post instructions on your job site for electrical incident first aid so that coworkers can provide effective assistance.

Heart attacks

The term "serious as a heart attack" really drives home how important it is to give immediate assistance if you suspect someone is having a heart attack. In the construction industry, heart attacks can be caused by an underlying health problem or result from an injury such as electrical shock. The signs of a heart attack include shortness of breath or difficulty breathing, crushing pain in the chest under the breast bone radiating down the left arm, or sudden jaw pain. The victim's skin may look pale or gray and they may complain about feeling nauseous, or begin perspiring or vomiting. Ask the person if they are on any medications or are allergic to aspirin, get them to sit down or recline, and loosen any tight clothing at their waist and neck. Do not let them walk or move around because this causes exertion, which will only increase the heart rate and the amount of oxygen that the heart needs to work. Call for help immediately and tell the responders that you suspect a heart attack. Many job sites have automatic external defibrillators, which are not complicated to use and come with step-by-step instructions. These do not require advanced training and are extremely effective. If there is no such device around, ask any other people present if they are trained in CPR. If the person stops breathing, and no one else is with you, it will be up to you to try to keep the person's heart pumping by pressing the palm of your hand on the lower section of the victim's breastbone in hard, rhythmic thrusts.

If the person remains conscious and doesn't stop breathing, stay with them until help arrives. Don't give the person any stimulants such as coffee or soda to drink, but you can give him/her an aspirin to chew. Aspirin works quickly, within 15 minutes, to prevent the formation of blood clots and decrease the risk for heart attack or a stroke. If possible, raise the person's legs up 12 to 18 inches to allow more blood to flow toward the heart.

Do not perform CPR unless the person becomes unconscious, stops breathing, or if you are unable to detect a heartbeat by holding your fingers against the left side of his/her neck just under the corner of the jaw.

CPR

Emergency cardiopulmonary resuscitation, CPR, is not as easy to perform as it looks on television. If you push too hard or in the wrong location on a person's chest you can crack ribs, puncture lungs, or rupture the diagram. Any of these complications can make it difficult or impossible for the person to begin breathing again. Ideally, CPR should be administered by someone who has been trained and has practiced the procedure. However, you may find yourself alone with someone who has stopped breathing as a result of an electrical shock or injury and be forced to try to help to the best of your ability. Call for help first, because the 911 operator can try to talk you through the CPR process. Here is what they are likely to advise you to do:

- Ask the person if they can hear you. Tell them to open their eyes and squeeze your hand.

- If you don't get a response, put one hand under the jaw and the other behind the head and tilt the head back gently. This should cause the person's mouth to open.

- Look at his/her chest to see if it is rising, and put your ear down to the mouth and listen for air escaping. If you can detect any breathing, turn the person over on to his/her left side and continue to check for breathing every 30 seconds.

- If the person stops breathing, provide "hands only" compressions by lifting his/her shirt and tracing an imaginary line between the nipples, then placing one hand horizontally along that line. Intertwine the fingers of your other hand between the fingers of the hand on the person's chest and press down with the palm of your hand until your arms are straight (Figure 11.16).

- Release only slightly, so that your elbows barely bend, and continue pressing up and down in this manner. You do not want to fully bend your arms, because it can exert too much pressure on the chest. Press down every second, and count the number of times you have compressed the person's chest until help arrives. This will keep you focused and help to keep you from panicking or slowing down.

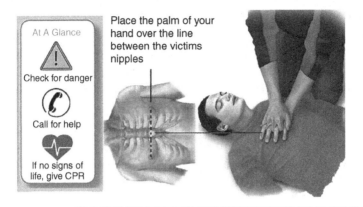

At A Glance

⚠️

Check for danger

📞

Call for help

If no signs of life, give CPR

Place the palm of your hand over the line between the victims nipples

Figure 11.16 Proper placement of your hands when performing chest compression can be the difference between helping and hurting a person in cardiac arrest.

- If the person begins to groan or move, stop compressions immediately and roll them onto their left side. Ask the person to squeeze your hand and assure them that help is on the way.

Accident reporting and investigation

Despite your best efforts, training, planning, and intentions, a job-related injury may still occur and you will need to know how to handle any mandatory reporting requirements. Depending on the type and severity of an accident or illness and your safety policy, you may be required to perform an accident investigation and file a report with OSHA, workers' compensation, and/or your insurance carrier.

An employer who truly has its employee's best interests in mind will always perform an accident investigation following a workplace incident. The main objectives are to eliminate hazards, reduce future construction accidents, and make work conditions safer for all workers. If you are the person who gets injured, try to remember that an accident investigation is not designed to make you look negligent or incompetent—on the contrary, it can protect your rights. If for some reason you have to pursue compensation legally, say because your injury was caused by someone else, an accident investigation report can document the facts about your injury.

An accident investigation is all about the facts. Details such as the date, time, and location will be listed, as well as the names of any witnesses. Your employment status, such as full or part-time, length of employment with your employer, job title (apprentice, helper, journeyman, master electrician), and rate of pay will also be noted. This information indicates your level of experience and financial compensation worth. The period of lost work time, days away from work, your diagnosis and prognosis, the form of treatment such as first aid, hospitalization, or surgery, and the severity of your injury will also be recorded. Specific details about your injury will also be documented. These include:

- The part of your body that was injured or affected, such as eye, neck, spine, knee, right or left arm or leg or hand or foot.

- The type of injury, from punctures, lacerations, or abrasions to muscular, skeletal, burns, or foreign body impact.

- The cause of the injury, such as impact from an object, falling, electrocution, slipping, tool malfunction, lifting, or the failure of another person to practice safe work methods.

- Factors that contributed to the incident, including inadequate supervision or training, equipment failure, failure to observe or employ safety controls, improper techniques, or inadequate or improper PPE.

- Corrective measure that can be used to avoid a similar incident in the future, such as improved enforcement or training, more frequent breaks or rotation of workers, replacement of tools, installation of more effective guards, use of lanyards, or additional or different PPE (Figure 11.17).

Mandatory reporting

Much of the accident report information will be needed to file a workers' compensation first report of injury or illness. This is required when an employee has lost one full day or a full shift of work due to an accident or work-related illness. Section 438 of the Workers' Compensation Act

PART of BODY INFURIED or AFFECTED						
☐ Skull, Scalp	☐ Jaw	☐ Abdomen	☐ Shoulder	☐ Wrist	☐ Knee	☐ Foot
☐ Eye	☐ Neck	☐ Back	☐ Upper Arm	☐ Hand	☐ Thigh	☐ Toe
☐ Nose	☐ Spine	☐ Pelvis	☐ Elbow	☐ Finger	☐ Lower Leg	☐ Ankle
☐ Mouth	☐ Chest	☐ Other Body Part	☐ Forearm	☐ Hip	☐ Other	

NATURE of INJURY or ILLNESS						
☐ Puncture	☐ Bruise, Contusion	☐ Skin Disorder	☐ Amputation	☐ Muscle Sprain	☐ Cumulative Trauma Disorder	
☐ Laceration	☐ Dislocation	☐ Burn	☐ Insect/Animal Bite	☐ Muscle Strain	☐ Irritation	
☐ Fracture	☐ Abrasion	☐ Respiratory	☐ Foreign Body	☐ Hernia	☐ Infection	
☐ Heat/Cold Stress	☐ Hearing Loss	☐ Chemical Exp.	☐ Other			

DISPOSITION	25. DIAGNOSIS	SEVERITY
☐ Days away from work # _____		☐ First Aid ☐ Medical Treatment
☐ Restricted work days # _____		☐ Lost Work Days ☐ Fatality
☐ Date returned to work # _____		☐ Other: Specify
Sent to: ☐ Doctor ☐ Hospital		

WHAT CONDITION of TOOLS, EQUIPMENT, or WORK AREA CONTRIBUTED TO INCIDENT?■Not Applicable

☐ Close Clearance/Congestion	☐ Floors/Work Surfaces	☐ Inadequate Housekeeping	☐ Defective Tools/Equipment/Vehicle
☐ Hazardous Placement	☐ Inadequate Ventilation	☐ Equipment Failure	☐ Illumination
☐ Inadequate Warning System	☐ Equipment/Workstation Design	☐ Inadequate Guards/Barrier	☐ Inadequate/Improper P.P.E.

WHAT CAUSED or INFLUENCED SUBSTANDARD CONDITIONS?   ■No Substandard Conditions

☐ Abuse or Misuse	☐ Inadequate Supervision	☐ Inadequate Purchasing	☐ Inadequate Engineering
☐ Inadequate Maintenance	☐ Inadequate Tools/Equip..Mat.	☐ Improper Work Surfaces	☐ Wear and Tear
☐ Lack of Knowledge/Training	☐ Improper Motivation	☐ Inadequate Capacity	☐ Lack of Skill

WHAT ACTION or INACTION CONTRIBUTED to the INCIDENT?   ■Not Applicable

☐ Failure to Make Secure	☐ Under Influence Drugs/Alcohol	☐ Failure to Warn/Signal	☐ Inadequate/Improper P. P. E. Use
☐ Nullified Safety/Control Devices	☐ Used Defective Equipment	☐ Horseplay/Distractive Active	☐ Operating at Improper Speed
☐ Used Equipment Improperly	☐ Improper Lifting	☐ Operating Procedure Deviation	
☐ Running/Rushing/Acting in Haste	☐ Improper Loading	☐ Unauthorized Actions	☐ Used Wrong Tool/Equipment
☐ Improper Technique	☐ Improper Position	☐ Servicing/Operating Equipment	

Figure 11.17 A sample section of an accident investigation shows the detailed information that is gathered to help improve safety measures and avoid future accidents.

requires employers to report work injuries to the Bureau of Workers' Compensation. Typically, an employer will submit this report via its workers' compensation insurance carrier, and has seven business days in which to file. As an injured worker it is vital that you report an injury or illness within 24 hours. There are several reasons for this, not the least of which is so that your employer can file its report within the mandatory filing period. Employers also have the right to require and determine medical care through their own company approved health care provider for the first 7 days following an injury. While you have the right to request a second opinion if you do not agree with their prognosis or treatment plan, most doctors chosen by employers have experience in work related injuries.

The quantity and frequency of workplace injuries affects an employer's workers' compensation experience modifier (MOD). This is a comparison of a company's actual loss experience to its expected loss experience over a period of 3 years. If you have higher-than-expected losses for your industry, your experience MOD will be greater than 1.00, and you will be charged additional insurance premiums. Money is a tremendous motivator, and this is a good example of how safety trainings and controls can pay off.

Any accident or incident that requires medical treatment other than first aid, or results in a restriction of normal work activities or days away from work has to be reported to OSHA. We've talked a lot in terms of injuries, but there are also a number of illnesses that fall under OSHA guidelines. Electricians can lose time from work due to heat stroke and heat exhaustion, frostbite, or exposure to blood-borne pathogens or hepatitis. For example, two electricians were working in a trench-burying conduit when sewage-contaminated liquid leaked into the ditch from an adjacent septic field. One of the electricians contracted Hepatitis A as a result of this workplace exposure.

Any case of worker injury or illness that requires lost time and on-going treatment must be reported to OSHA. Employers are required to maintain accurate records of work-related deaths, injuries, and illnesses other than minor injuries requiring only first aid treatment that do not involve medical treatment, loss of consciousness, restriction of work or motion, or transfer to another job. OSHA Form 301, Injury and Illness Incident Report, contains much of the same information as an accident investigation report. This information is used by OSHA for data collection to assist in the development of safety and health programs and standard evaluation (Figure 11.18).

The details regarding workplace injuries are entered on an OSHA 300 form, A Summary of Work-Related Injuries and Illnesses. All of the log entries are compiled on this form. You must enter each recordable injury or illness on the OSHA 300 Log and 301 Incident Report within seven calendar days of receiving information that a recordable injury or illness has occurred.

According to Public Law 91-596 and 29 CFR 1904, OSHAs recordkeeping rule, you must keep these OSHA 300 forms on file for 5 years.

Case number from the *Log* _____ *(Transfer the case number from the Log after you record the case.)*

Date of injury or illness _____ / _____ / _____

Time employee began work _____ AM / PM

Time of event _____ AM / PM ☐ Check if time cannot be determined

---

What was the employee doing just before the incident occurred? Describe the activity, as well as the tools, equipment, or material the employee was using. Be specific. *Examples:* "climbing a ladder while carrying roofing materials"; "spraying chlorine from hand sprayer"; "daily computer key-entry."

What happened? Tell us how the injury occurred. *Examples:* "When ladder slipped on wet floor, worker fell 20 feet"; "Worker was sprayed with chlorine when gasket broke during replacement"; "Worker developed soreness in wrist over time."

What was the injury or illness? Tell us the part of the body that was affected and how it was affected; be more specific than "hurt," "pain," or sore." *Examples:* "strained back"; "chemical burn, hand"; "carpal tunnel syndrome."

What object or substance directly harmed the employee? *Examples:* "concrete floor"; "chlorine"; "radial arm saw."

If the employee died, when did death occur? Date of death _____ / _____ / _____

Figure 11.18 Many employers neglect to complete OSHA form 301 because they believe an accident report is all that is required of them.

In addition to mandatory reporting, your insurance carrier may have independent requirements for reporting accidents or worker illness. One example is commercial vehicle insurance carriers, which may require you to report any accidents involving a company vehicle within 24 hours. You may also be required to provide proof that employees do not use company tools, equipment, or vehicles for personal use.

It may all seem like too much paperwork and inconvenience for you to handle, but all of these prevention and reporting requirements are in place to help protect employers and their workers. Being an electrician is a dangerous occupation. Don't expose yourself to unnecessary safety risks or exposure for lawsuits, outrageous insurance premiums, or fines (Figure 11.19). Better safe than sorry needs to be your motto (Figure 11.00).

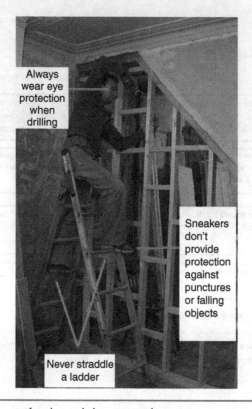

Always wear eye protection when drilling

Sneakers don't provide protection against punctures or falling objects

Never straddle a ladder

Figure 11.19   Three safety hazards by one worker.

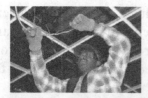

Proactive Measures to Reduce Injury

Minimize Awkward Postures
Avoid pressure on palms, wrists, elbows, and knees
Select the correct tool handle orientation based upon worksurface height/orientation
Use mechanical lift assists and carts
Use proper lifting techniques when lifting

Figure 11.00   Ergonomic Safety Fast Facts.

(Continued)

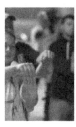

Benfits of Stetching

Increases flexibility/elasticity of muscles
Increases circulation to warm the muscles, improving mental alertness, reducing fatigue
Decreases muscle tension and stress

When to Stretch

Prior to starting your day
During short breaks (at least once per hour)
After breaks or lunch to prevent fatigue
If tension or stress is apparent
After a lengthy task duration or an extended awkward posture

Proper stretching techniques:

Relax and breathe normally. Do not hold your breath.
Hold each stretch for a count of 15, or as long as comfort is maintained.
Use gentle, controlled motions. Do not bounce!
Keep the knees slightly bent for better balance.
Stretch until a mild tension is felt, then relax.
Stretch by how you feel and not by how far you can go.

Figure 11.00—Cont'd.

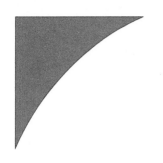

Chapter 12

Safe Work Practices

Chapter Outline

283

Tradesmen invest a lot of time and money to acquire the skills necessary to become proficient at their jobs so they can earn top dollar for their work. Business owners spend a lot of money building and promoting their company and making their business profitable. One of the key work practices that can either make or break a company or individual is safety. Safety is not a theory or good intention, it is the resulting outcome of specific actions. Safety is what you get if things are done properly and events go as planned. Electricity is intrinsically hazardous and demands those who work with or around it to plan for and guard against possible exposure. You have the right to leave work everyday in the same state of health as when you arrived to start your day. Customers expect electrical installations that will operate without risk of damage to their property or injury to the people who inhabit it. When you combine and comply with standards and regulations that have been established to minimize electrical hazards, you maximize your profitability and personal well-being.

Electricians who work safely have higher productivity and less worker turnover, lost time, and material waste. Contractors who focus on safe work practices have lower overhead costs, insurance costs, labor costs, and higher profit margins. On the other hand, contractors with negative safety records are viewed as dangerous and uncaring by their employees, resulting in higher labor turnover. Turnovers add to the costs for this type of contractor, who ends up with increased costs for training new employees over and over again. The contractor may settle for less skilled electricians or helpers, which increases production costs. Research has shown that newer workers have a higher rate of accidents on the job. This is usually because they do things like hurry to prove they can meet deadlines, or because they are unfamiliar with the equipment used or job site conditions in general. In the long run, it is less expensive to encourage and enforce safe working practices than it is to ignore them.

Safety conscious employer interviews

As a business owner or manager, you can begin saving your company money from the moment you interview a potential employee by determining their skill level. Begin your evaluation of their ability to perform the type of work you need them to do by using an employment application with a physical abilities section that targets their physical condition. Simple questions could include "Have you ever":

- Suffered from hearing problems or hearing loss?

- Suffered from visual problems or eye diseases?

- Had back problems, back pain, or back injuries or operations?

- Had foot or knee problems, injuries, or operations?

- Have you ever been a patient in a hospital for any reason? If YES, have them provide an explanation of dates and reasons for hospitalizations.

- Lost time from work in the past year for any reason? If YES, have them provide dates and explanations for the causes.

- Do you smoke cigarettes? Add a note that some job sites may be in smoke-free locations, or if your company prohibits smoking on company property or in company vehicles, add that note to this section as well.

These types of health situations can hamper a potential employee's ability to perform their job at an optimum level. Beyond these types of general health questions, you will want to know that a worker possesses the skill level required for the position you are hiring. The best way to establish this is to provide a separate sheet that lists the trade skills and physical requirements of the specific position you are hiring. For example,

- Study blueprints and schematics and determine methods, materials, and equipment needed to complete the work project. Perform material take-offs and complete permit applications, including confined space.

- Connect wires to plugs, switches, controls, light fixtures, appliances, motors, breaker panels, and switchboards. Pull wire through conduit.

- Test installations to ensure continuity of the circuit and the compatibility and safety of all components using test equipment such as an ohmmeter, ampmeter, voltmeter, etc.

- Perform the duties of the job site qualified worker by demonstrating knowledge and training on safe work methods for energized work, lockout/tagout, hazard analysis, short-circuit studies, and arc flash/blast boundaries.

- Proven knowledge of applicable PPE to meet OSHA requirements.

- Measure, cut, bend, thread, assemble, and install electrical conduit, junction, switch, outlet boxes, and switch boards using hand tools and equipment such as mechanical drills, cutters, benders, and threaders.

- Inspect and evaluate electrical equipment to ensure that it operates efficiently and safely; determine whether equipment and new installations meet requirements of the National Electrical Code.

- Assist in training lower-level electricians. Provide instruction and training in the proper methods, processes, and safe work practices necessary to carry out electrician assignments.

- Develop plans and estimates for electrical projects; includes determining time, equipment, and human and material resources needed to complete the work.

- Ability to lift 75 pounds and work overhead from a ladder or scaffold.

- Experience wearing a respirator and working in confined spaces.

- A valid driver's license with no violations within the past 5 years.

- A reliable means of transportation.

- No felony convictions.

On your employment application, include a statement that the applicant has read and understands the job description and is not aware of any reasons or restrictions that would prohibit him/her from performing these duties. These questions allow you to compare any potential applicant's risks or areas that would require training or special accommodations.

There are, however, a number of questions that you are not permitted to ask during an interview. It is illegal to specifically ask an applicant's age, country of national origin, religion, marital or family status, or if they have ever incurred a work-related injury. Be especially mindful during the course of a comfortable interview not to ask seemingly innocuous interview questions that could be illegal, such as:

- What arrangements are you able to make for childcare while you work?

- How old are your children?

- When did you graduate from high school?

- Are you a U.S. citizen?

- What does your wife do for a living?

- Where did you live while you were growing up?

- Will you need personal time for particular religious holidays?

- Are you comfortable working for a female boss?

- There appears to be a large disparity between your age and that of the position's coworkers. Is this a problem for you?

- How long do you plan to work until you retire?

- Have you ever filed for workers' compensation?

Pre-employment physical exams

Employment physical examinations are conducted to assess an applicant's ability to perform the duties required of a position. To protect against discrimination in hiring, the physical examination should be required after a job is offered. Physical Ability Tests Physical ability tests measure the physical ability of an applicant to perform a particular task or the strength of specific muscle groups, as well as strength and stamina in general. Many employers contract with companies or medical facilities that specialize in these tests. Our company used a firm that performed thorough and unique physical assessment tests that demonstrated applicants' skills and safe work practices. For example, the company had a platform with several tiers at its testing site and a container of various PPE such as gloves, kneepads, goggles, and earplugs. Applicants were shown where the PPE was and were asked to perform a number of activities such as: go up and down stairs, squat down and pick up lengths of #1 AWG wire and place them on a shelf overhead, carry a 75 pound roll of wire for a specific distance, climb and stand on a ladder for 10 minutes while reaching up and repeatedly popping up a ceiling tile, use a screwdriver to attach different types of screws into a piece of wood, lift and operate a power saw (without a blade), and even crawl through a piece of corrugated sewer pipe (Figure 12.1).

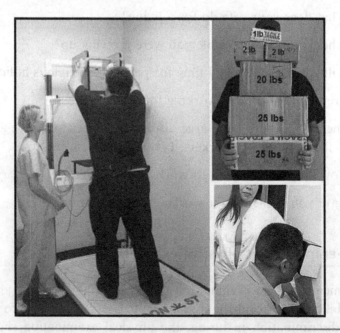

Figure 12.1 Physical ability tests can be used to measure a potential employee's stamina, strength, vision, and knowledge of personal protective equipment requirements.

Not only did the tester measure the applicant's physical ability to perform these common tasks, but it was also noted whether the potential employee used applicable PPE. We were amazed at how many applicants never used any of the PPE during their testing. If an applicant doesn't think about putting on goggles to lift ceiling tiles, earplugs to run a saw, or kneepads or gloves to crawl on their hands and knees during a test, they are not intuitively safety conscious. It is one thing to possess the basic electrical skills required to do the job. It is another to have the physical capability to perform them day in and day out in a safe manner that protects an employee from harm. By focusing on safety from the first interview, an employer can increase the odds of hiring and keeping healthy, productive, safe electricians.

> You can also provide a safety quiz for applicants to complete that will help you gauge their understanding of issues such as PPE and OSHA safe work standards. This shows potential employees that you are focused on safety and provides you with a tangible idea of their safe work practice experience.

Employee safety concerns

As an employee, you have the right to work in a safe environment and to have an employer who values your health and well-being as both a worker and a person. A business manager is not the only party who should ask safety-related questions during your interview process. You can learn a lot about your potential employer by asking a few questions of your own. Not just the typical inquiry about paid sick leave and health benefits, but questions about the employer's safety practices. For example, you could ask if the company has an injury and illness prevention program, or if they provide safety training on specific equipment, such as forklifts, that you may need to use as part of your job with the company.

Employee safety rights

Once you are working for a company, you need to keep your safety high on your priority list. Remember that OSHAs primary purpose is to establish and encourage workplace safety standards that are designed to save lives, prevent workplace injuries and illnesses, and protect the health of workers. This means that as a worker, you have specific rights under OSHA. For example, you are allowed to request and receive information concerning OSHA rules and regulations so that you can become familiar with them. These regulations include conducting mandatory measuring or monitoring of toxic substances on your job site, and all emergency procedures.

> You also have the right to receive training that is required by OSHA standards. For example, if your employer wants you to move materials from delivery trucks using a forklift, you have the right and responsibility to request training and certification on forklift operation. Without proper training, you pose a safety risk not only to yourself, but to others as well.

You have the right to refuse to perform work assigned to you if you reasonably believe that a hazardous condition exists that poses a genuine threat of serious injury or death. If you request that your employer correct this type of condition and they fail to do so, you have the right to place a confidential safety complaint to OSHA concerning workplace conditions and to receive a follow-up inspection or investigation. You are permitted to participate in an OSHA walk-around, regardless of whether or not it is related to a complaint you filed. You also have the right to learn the results of any OSHA inspection that takes place at your company's site, as well as to participate in OSHA consultation services and be advised of those results (Figure 12.2).

Realistically, OSHA statistics gauge non-safety. When you really think about it, all OSHA measurements are based on the failure of the safety process—fatalities, lost workdays, recordable injuries, and the number of workdays lost per injury. For example, OSHA statistics show that 90% of fatalities occur in four categories—someone caught between objects, struck by objects, electrocution, and falls. OSHA does not provide figures on how many employees at any given company have not been involved in an accident or who are alive and well. OSHA views accidents as preventable and incidents that can be avoided with the proper safety training, precaution, and common sense. Safety, under the OSHA statistics approach, is measured by the occurrence of fatalities or events, known as mishaps or near misses. When a negative event happens, it manifests

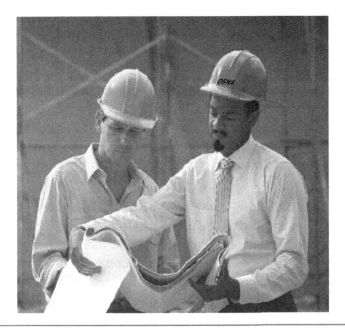

Figure 12.2 You have the right to be an informed employee and to participate in OSHA inspections at your job site.

itself on the job site, leaving a trace to be measured. Most companies do not hand out rewards to workers who have not been hurt over time. So as an employee, the true measure of your dedication to safe-work practices is demonstrated by the fact that you leave work everyday uninjured. That statistic should be enough to make any of us happy.

Material safety data sheets

Safety precautions involve more than just being mindful of your surroundings and wearing proper PPE. There is a book that has to be kept on all construction sites, which, in my experience, few electricians ever open or peruse because they don't think it contains anything that applies to them. This is the book or folder that contains material safety data sheets. Material safety data sheets, known in the industry as MSDS, must be developed for all hazardous chemicals used in the workplace, and must list the hazardous chemicals that are found in a product in quantities of 1% or greater, or 0.1% or greater if the chemical is a carcinogen.

MSDS information is mandatory under OSHA paragraph (g) of 29 CFR 1910.1200.

The MSDS is a detailed informational document prepared by the manufacturer of a hazardous chemical that describes the physical and chemical properties of the product. The MSDS contains useful information such as a chemical's flash point, toxicity, storage guidelines, and procedures for spills and leaks.

The chemicals that pose a potential health hazard present on a job site could be as simple as cleaning products, bleach, paint, waterproofing products, and soldering flux. Used independently and with adequate ventilation, these products are safe to use; however, many products used in the construction industry pose serious health risks if combined with other chemical products. One of the factors listed on an MSDS is chemical reactivity. This is the ability of a material to undergo a chemical change. A chemical reaction can occur under conditions such as heating, burning, contact with other chemicals, or even exposure to light. Here is an example that happened to one electrician. He was running wires for a remodeling job in a dormitory bathroom when he tugged on the wire and knocked over a container of bleach that was on the top of the toilet. He wiped up the bleach with a rag and then sprayed a bottle of cleaner he found in the site trailer on the area to remove the bleach residue. He closed the bathroom door, replaced the bottle of cleaner and then returned to finish his work. When he opened the door and went back into the bathroom to finish his work, he became dizzy and nauseous. What happened? The industrial spray cleaner actually contained hydrochloric acid. When this combined with the chemicals that make up bleach, a toxic gas chlorine was produced and trapped behind the closed bathroom door. Chlorine gas, also known as bertholite, has been used as a chemical weapon since World War 1. When chlorine is inhaled, it reacts with the water in the mucus in your lungs and forms the irritant hydrochloric acid, which can be lethal. All of this happened because the electrician never stopped to check the MSDS to see if the cleaner he grabbed could chemically react with the substance he was cleaning up.

The physical characteristics that are listed on the MSDS include whether a material is corrosive under any conditions. A corrosive material can corrode metals and cause metal containers or structural materials to become weak and eventually to leak or collapse.

The can also burn or destroy human tissues on contact and can cause permanent scarring or blindness. An example of a corrosive product that you have probably used if you have ever had to solder any materials is flux, which contains phosphoric acid. Rust remover also contains phosphoric acid.

One of the important items of information provided on the MSDS is the exposure limit for chemical compounds. An exposure limit is the concentration of a chemical in the workplace air that most people can be exposed to without experiencing harmful effects. Some products list this exposure as the short-term exposure limit (STEL). This is the average concentration to which workers can be exposed for a short period (usually 15 minutes) without experiencing irritation, long-term or irreversible tissue damage, or reduced alertness. Another part of the data to pay attention to is any explosive limits that may be listed. Explosive limits specify the concentration range of a material in the air that will burn or explode in the presence of an ignition source such as a spark or a flame. The MSDS will also list how chemicals in the product enter your body, such as topically, as a vapor or gas, or if swallowed (Figure 12.3).

Information included in a material safety data sheet needs to be available to help you select safe products, understand the potential health and physical hazards of a chemical, and understand how to respond effectively to exposure situations. Each sheet lists the label name of the product, the chemical and common names of the substance, all ingredients, and any specific hazards such as chemical reactions. Additionally, there will be a statement of any ingredients that are known carcinogens. As you can see, the safety aspects of material safety data sheets are something that you should become familiar with before you use any substance that contains chemicals.

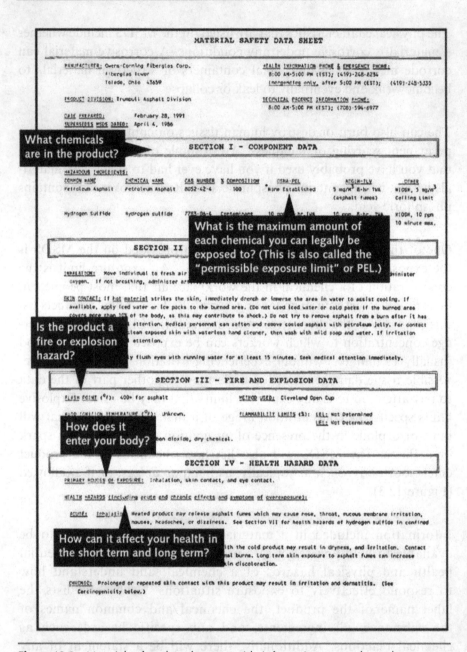

Figure 12.3 Material safety data sheets provide information on any hazardous aspects of a product's chemical makeup.

Workers' compensation facts

Almost every electrician has heard about workers' compensation and knows that it pays for medical expenses if someone gets hurt on the job. As an employee, there may be a number of facts about workers' compensation that you are not aware of. For example, your employer's workers' compensation insurance company gets to choose your initial medical provider. If you have to be referred to a medical specialist, the insurance company gets to choose that particular doctor as well. Many workers' compensation insurance companies will reimburse you for gas used driving to and from your doctor appointments. Once you are examined by the doctor, your injury will be classified as either a temporary total disability (TTD) or a temporary partial disability (TPD).

A TTD means that you are currently medically unable to perform any of your pre-injury work activities. Temporary partial disabled employees are able to return to work with doctor-imposed physical restrictions that prevent them from performing all of the duties of their pre-injury position. Don't let these terms intimidate you. For example, if you are a journeyman electrician and you are going to be on crutches for 6 weeks because you broke your ankle, then you are not able to perform any of your duties for that period of time. You can't carry tools, operate equipment, pull wire, install fixtures or trim, or even safely navigate your way through a construction site. You are temporarily totally disabled. On the other hand, if you broke a finger you could still carry tools, move safely around a job site, and maybe install trim materials such as outlet and switch covers. A doctor would probably allow you to work with restrictions such as no overhead work, or equipment operation and so you are only temporarily partially disabled. These types of injuries should heal without permanent complications and you should be back on the job full-time soon enough. However, if you have incurred a back, neck, or head injury you may suffer from physical impairments that will last a lifetime (Figure 12.4).

An impairment rating is a way for a doctor to rate the severity of your injury and is provided at the end of your medical treatment. If your doctor assigns an impairment rating that exceeds an established percentage, say 20%, you may be entitled to permanent total disability

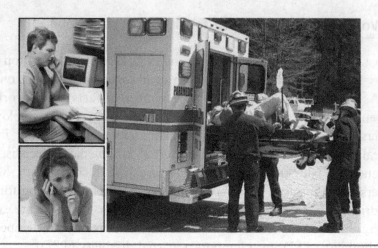

Figure 12.4 A workplace injury means that you will lose time and full wages from your job, not to mention the worry and burden to your family. Safe work practices will minimize your risk of being injured.

benefits. This means that you will probably not be able to perform all of the duties of your job without pain or risking additional injury. Situations such as these will require you to re-think your vocation and, if possible, change jobs to a career that is less physically demanding.

Let's assume that you will be able to return to work after a period of time completely healed. In the meantime, you will be collecting workers' compensation payments for your wages. In my experience, most electricians seem to think that they will receive 100% of their hourly wage, based on what they were making when they got hurt. I have actually had electricians who had just finished working overtime ask me why their payments were less than what they brought home in their last check. The answer is that while your work accident compensation is based on your average weekly wage, known as your AWW, it is not determined by your last or highest full-time check. The AWW is calculated by averaging your wages during the 13-week period immediately preceding that date of your accident or injury. So that overtime that you just started is only a portion of your wage base. If you have been injured before you worked a full 13 weeks, your employer can use wages from another employee that has worked 13 weeks and is employed in the same position that you hold. As you can see, being injured and on workers' compensation is not your ticket to easy street and a free check every other week. While workers' compensation exists to make sure that you receive some reparation for your wages while you are recuperating, the best way to ensure that your livelihood is not affected is to stay safe and unharmed while you are at work.

Employer workers compensation facts

An employer's workers' compensation MOD rating is based on a number of factors, including the cost of workers' injuries over a period of time. This means that fewer injuries directly equates to lower insurance premiums. It can also be the difference between being awarded contracts and not being eligible to bid on a job. Many large companies and institutions, such as colleges, will only accept bids from contractors with a workers' compensation MOD below a set level. Your MOD can save you money in premiums and earn you money by providing you the ability to bid on a wide-range of projects. For these reasons, it is important for an employer to understand what data is used to establish a MOD rating.

When a MOD is analyzed, employers can see a history of their claims. The data includes the cost of the injuries by employee name, and the number of modification points attributed to each injury. If there has been an increase in premiums for the current year, the costs will be broken down by specific employee injuries. The cumulative increased premium cost over a 3-year period will also be shown.

Workers compensation costs

Job classification is the main factor determining the cost of your premiums. Electricians, roofers, and construction tradesmen who work around heavy equipment have the highest risks of severe injury, and office workers have the lowest risk. So it is up to you, as an employer, to ensure that you keep your premiums as realistic as you can to control costs.

When you assign job titles, duties, and categories, it is important to consider how these factors will affect the premium to be assessed for each employee. Each work classification is assigned a workers' compensation code and costs are based on the number of employees you have in each code. For example, there is a code for electrical wiring—within buildings (#5190), a different code for electricians who work only with low voltage systems such as communication systems or alarms (#7605) and then one code for electrician, electrical assistant, electrician senior level, electrician supervisor, and electrician senior supervisor (#3179). There is a separate code for laborers. Electrician helpers or apprentices would be considered a code #3179, unless the majority of their duties classify them as a laborer. The rate for a low voltage electrician is approximately half that of the standard electrician class. The best way to determine the premiums for each code is to consult your workers' compensation insurance carrier for an explanation of the duties associated with the various codes.

The basic workers' compensation rates for each job classification are set by each individual state and are based on payroll costs. When paying an employee time and a half for overtime, you may only have to report the regular wages, decreasing the amount of payroll that determines your insurance premiums. Many insurance carriers will quote you lower rates if your company implements pre-claim and post-claim programs. Some of these risk management measures include the following practices.

Return to work programs

Establishing a return to work program allows an employee to come back to work in a number of capacities. An employee can return to work part time or to a position that accommodates any restrictions they may have. Let's think about the type of jobs and duties that are performed by a typical electrical contracting firm that do not require a lot of physical activity. Someone has to estimate work, perform material take-offs, and prepare bids and presentations. Orders need to be processed and expedited, deliveries need to be received and checked, and inventory such as fittings, covers, lightbulbs, and other lightweight items need to be taken to job sites. These are all tasks that an electrician who is not yet 100% can perform.

Modified duties are another way to get employees back to work. For example, an employee who is restricted from working on a ladder or overhead could install outlets and switches. If the same employee cannot stand for long periods of time, he/she could sit on a stool to trim out the receptacles. Rising workers' compensation costs are primarily due to the increased use of benefits and longer durations of disability. The more time an employee spends on disability, the more wage replacement and medical services increase in cost. By getting employees off workers' compensation quickly, you reduce the duration and expense of their claim. This benefits employees as well, by getting them back into the swing of regular working hours and including them in aspects of the business that they may not have experienced before.

Analyzing previous claims

Look for a pattern to claims. Do some locations or areas in your business have more claims than others? Determine the reason why. You can use your accident investigation forms, first injury reports, and OSHA Form 301 Injury and Illness Incident Report to analyze repetitive injuries or site locations. This will help you to identify areas within your company that require specific or more frequent safety training. Perhaps you need to provide additional training to a site supervisor or change the type of equipment you have been using. Once you have identified hazard or risk issues and begin targeted safety, you can provide documentation to your workers' compensation insurance carrier as proof that you are taking steps to reduce injuries and illness within your company. The result should be fewer claims and by reducing the number of workers' compensation claims your business safety record will improve. This means you are a much better risk to an insurance company, making it more likely they will give you better rates in the long run (Figure 12.5).

You can also implement a number of pre-claims programs aimed at preventing accidents and provide your insurance carrier with this information as well. Document every form of safety training that your company provides, including safety talks, regular safety checks,

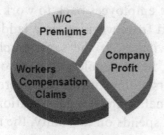
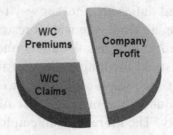

2005 Profile of a Electrical Contracting Firm in Virginia prior to implementation of Workplace Safety Protocols. Top two injury categories were: Skeletal/Musular such as back injuries and broken bones, and Tissue Damage such as burns, eye injuries, cuts, and electrical shocks (non-fatal).

2009 Profile of the same Electrical Contracting Firm following three consecutive years of implemnating regular Safety Trainings, Incentive programs, Supervisor trainings, Pre-employment Ability Testing, and Modified Return To Work programs.

Figure 12.5 This graphic illustrates how reducing workers' compensation claims lowers premiums and results in higher overall profits.

equipment service and maintenance records, revisions to your company's safety manual, and period site inspections. If your company offers a safety incentive program, be sure to provide your insurance carrier with a list of the number of employees who have received acknowledgements or rewards for their safe work practices. Additionally, you will want to give your carrier a list of all specific safety programs offered over the course of a year, such as respirator training, first aid and CPR courses attended by your employees, forklift or scissor lift trainings and certifications, and any preferred doctors or medical clinics that you use for employee assessment and treatment. You will also want to detail any corrective measures your company has taken based on your safety analysis procedures, as well as improvements that exist as a result (Figure 12.6).

The right tools for safety

Using the right tool for the job is a simple and extremely effective safe work practice. This can be as basic as choosing the correct type of saw blade for the material you need to cut. Taking the time to match the

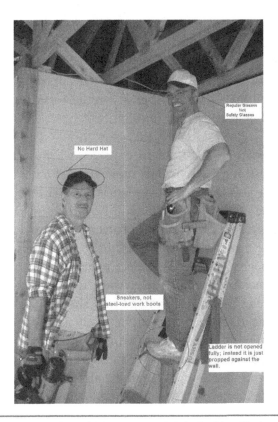

Figure 12.6 A spot inspection of this contractor's job site identified a number of safety infractions. The supervisor snapped this photo and then marked-up and posted the picture on the job site as a reminder for all employees to think about safety and practice safe work methods.

blade to the material means it will take you less time in the long run to cut a material and decrease the risk of the saw kicking back, skipping across the material, or becoming bound up and damaged.

As an electrician, your meter is one of your best safety tools. We have already discussed the importance of making sure that circuits and equipment are de-energized before you start working on them. The first way to confirm that no electricity is present is to use an ammeter because it specifically measures the electric current in a circuit. To measure larger currents, a resistor called a shunt is placed in parallel with the meter. Most of the current flows through the shunt, and only a small fraction flows through the meter. This allows the meter to measure large currents. If you detect current where there should be none, you will want to determine the source of electricity. Your voltmeter should be used for measuring the electrical potential difference between two points in an electric circuit. Of course, you could use a combination multimeter that will give you the versatility of measuring voltage, current, and resistance in ohms.

There are a number of factors to consider when you decide which meter type to use for a particular application. First of all, the meter needs to have a voltage capability that is at least equal to or greater than the voltage of the circuit you will be measuring. The meter also needs to have internal short circuit protection to ensure that if it fails internally it will not cause a short circuit to appear at the measuring probes. This means you should select a meter with resistance leads or internal fuses. Additionally, you want to choose a meter that is capable of reading the lowest voltage that should be present from all sources, such as back-feed current as well as the normal voltage. Impedance is the final aspect for you to take into consideration. You need the meter to be capable of measuring current that is couple to the circuit and has a high enough circuit impedance so that it doesn't load the circuit and reduce the system voltage to what only appears to be a safe level (Figure 12.7).

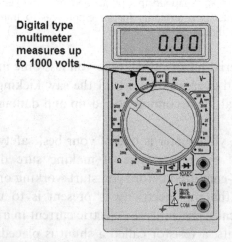

Figure 12.7 A typical example of a multimeter that is capable of measuring voltage up 1000 V rather than a cap limit of only 600 V.

The IEC 61010 is a standard that defines the usage of various types of meters by establishing categories based on voltage and applications. For example, a category I meter should be used for electronics with inherently low energy. This would be equipment that is cord-connected and has built-in transient suppression in the equipment or supply. Category II meters should be used for single-phase receptacle-connected equipment, such as portable tools, branch circuits, and appliances. Indoor lighting circuits, motors, switchgear, and industrial applications including bus and feeders should be measured using a category III meter. These are designed for three-phase or single-phase distribution systems that are isolated for main utility power supplies by transformers or other surge protection. The final group is category IV meters which are used for current that is directly connected to utility circuits and feeders, such as service entrance equipment and power utility service meters. Additionally, Section 110.6(D)(1)(e) of NFPA 70E-2009 requires workers to be trained in the use of voltage detectors and understand the readings and settings of the metering equipment.

If you need to work on energized circuits, you will need to use high-voltage tools that are designed to insulate against current. A hot stick electrically insulates you from energized conductors and provides a physical separation from the device being operated to reduce the chance of burns that may result from electrical arcing if there is a malfunction of the device being operated. Fiberglass hot sticks are used by electric utility workers on live-line work or by commercial electrical contractors. For utility workers, a hot stick allows them to perform operations on power lines without de-energizing them or when the state of the power line is not yet known. This is essential because some operations, such as opening or closing combination fuse/switches, must occasionally be performed on an energized line. Additionally, after a fault has occurred, the exact state of a line may not be certain and utility workers must treat the line as though it were energized until it can be proven that it is not. Depending on the tool you attach to the end of a hot stick, you can test for voltage, tighten nuts and bolts, open and close switches, replace fuses, or lay insulating sleeves on wires without exposing yourself or a crew to a large risk of electric shock (Figure 12.8).

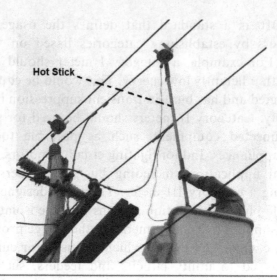

Figure 12.8 Insulated hot sticks provide insulation and separation between an electrician and an energized circuit.

A hot stick and any tools attached to it need to be wiped clean and stored so that it is protected from moisture. A hot stick with a defect, such as a surface rupture, needs to be repaired or replaced. American Society for Testing and Materials (ASTM) Standard F 711 specifies stringent requirements for hot sticks. Industry regulations for hot stick testing include IEEE Standard 978-1984 and OSHA Standard 1910.269 (j)(2)(iii) which require that live-line tools used for primary employee protection must be removed from service, inspected, and electrically tested every 2 years.

Electrical protective gloves

High voltage gloves are a form of PPE that is required for employees who work in close proximity to live electrical current. OSHAs Electrical Protective Equipment Standard (29 CFR 1910.137) provides the design guidelines and in-service care and use requirements for electrical-insulating gloves and sleeves as well as insulating blankets, matting, covers, and line hoses (Figure 12.9).

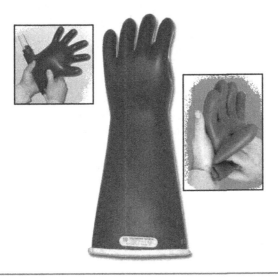

Figure 12.9   High voltage gloves must be rated and tested for safety in accordance with OSHA and ASTM standards.

Electrical protective gloves are categorized by the level of voltage protection they provide. Voltage protection is broken down into the following classes:

- Class 0—Maximum use voltage of 1000 V AC/proof tested to 5000 V AC.

- Class 1—Maximum use voltage of 7500 V AC/proof tested to 10,000 V AC.

- Class 2—Maximum use voltage of 17,000 V AC/proof tested to 20,000 V AC.

- Class 3—Maximum use voltage of 26,500 V AC/proof tested to 30,000 V AC.

- Class 4—Maximum use voltage of 36,000 V AC/proof tested to 40,000 V AC.

Once the gloves are issued, OSHA requires that they be maintained in a safe, reliable condition. This means that high voltage gloves must be inspected for any damage before each day's use, and immediately following any incident that may have caused them to be damaged.

This test method is described in the ASTM section F 496, Specification for In-Service Care of Insulating Gloves and Sleeves. Basically, the glove is filled with air, manually or by an inflator, and then checked for leakage.

The easiest way to detect leakage is by listening for air escaping or holding the glove against your cheek to feel air releasing.

OSHA recognizes that gloves meeting ASTM D 120-87, Specification for Rubber Insulating Gloves, and ASTM F 496, Specification for In-Service Care of Insulating Gloves and Sleeves, meet its requirements. In addition to daily testing, OSHA requires periodic electrical tests for electrical protective equipment and ASTM F 496 specifies that gloves must be electrically retested every 6 months. Many power utility companies will test gloves and hot sticks for a reasonable fee.

Electrical safety tips

Don't get so focused on the big hazards, like arc blast, that you overlook the more common safety risks for electricians. For example, over 40 workers died last year from falls after they stepped or sat on skylights that then broke under their weight. To prevent falls like this, follow the same OSHA regulations that you would for open roof work and install guard rails around every skylight before starting work. Also, putting safety netting underneath any type of roof openings during construction can save lives.

Not many electricians would risk standing knee deep in water or in the pouring rain while they are testing electrical circuits. But not everyone thinks about the dangers of something as basic as damp conditions. Suppose it stopped raining an hour ago, but the ground or concrete is still wet, or it is humid and your clothes are damp. These are the times when you need to either avoid using electric tools or wear protective equipment such as insulated rubber gloves and boots. In hot weather, high humidity, or even foggy conditions, remind yourself to towel off frequently, because believe it or not, even perspiration can be conductive. Dry your hands carefully before handling flexible cords and equipment that's plugged in, and if possible, turn off the electricity before you start working. Be cautious also not to run extension cords through damp or wet areas, especially if you are working on a ladder or scaffolding. Even a small shock could cause you to lose your balance. Additionally, any form of temporary wiring should only be used during remodeling, maintenance, repair, demolition and similar activities. Temporary wiring for 15- and 20-ampere 125-volt single-phase receptacles should also include ground-fault circuit interrupters.

And don't forget to make sure that every work site and company vehicle is equipped with a first aid kit to meet OSHA regulation 1910.151(b) and the ANSI Z308.1-2003 requirement. Basic first aid kits should include the basics, such as tweezers, knuckle fabric bandages, a gauze roll and pads, antiseptic wipes, an instant cold compress, and scissors. Construction site first aid kits should also include one blood bourn pathogen kit and mouth covers or protectors in case mouth-to-mouth resuscitation needs to be performed. It is an added bonus to include burn and antibiotic cream, aspirin, ibuprofen, and acetaminophen.

Trenches

Electricians don't usually have to work in trenches often enough to be familiar with safety protocols for this type of risk. Most workers know to call ahead of time and have underground utilities located and marked before they begin digging to install conduit or conduct repairs. But did you know that excavations and trenches that are more than 4 feet deep must have proper sloping and shoring, and a safe exit such as a ramp or ladder within 25 feet of every worker. Beyond that, trenches that are 5 feet or deeper must be inspected daily by a qualified environmental health and safety professional. Any excavated dirt, material, or other objects must be kept at least 2 feet from a trench opening. Additionally, no one is allowed to work on the sides of sloped or benched excavations above other employees unless the worker in the trench is protected from falling material. You also need to station a top person outside the trench to detect moving ground and warn workers to leave the trench. As you can see, working in a trench requires much more than just the knowledge of how to bend and run the conduit that goes in it.

Any excavating under the base or footing of a foundation or wall requires a support system designed by a registered professional engineer.

Code compliant safety

By now you have probably figured out that working safely demands planning, common sense, and a strong understanding of the safety codes that apply to the task you need to perform. Before you pick up your wire cutters or screwdriver, you should take the time to assess the site conditions and related factors such as power supplies, equipment, and tools that will be involved in your work for the day. If you are unsure of any of the codes that will apply to the type of work you are about to perform, here are a few cross-referenced codes for you to familiarize yourself with.

- Hazards: Have the hazards been identified and have you and those who will be working with you been trained in those hazards? See OSHA 1910.332(A) and NFPA 110.6(A). Will you be working in a hazardous location and has the hazard classification been determined? See OSHA 1910.307(a), NFPA 440.3(A), and NEC 500.5.

- De-energizing power: Has the current been de-energized and tested to confirm that all power has been disconnected? For de-energizing requirements, see OSHA 1910.333(a)(1), NFPA 70E 120.2, and NEC Table 110.26(A)(1). For lockout/tagout requirements see OSHA 29 CFR 1910.147 and NFPA 120.2.

- Energized Equipment: Would de-energizing power create a hazard? For regulations on working with energized equipment, see OSHA 1910.33(a)(2). NFPA 70E Article 110.8(B)(1) requires an electrical hazard analysis before work is performed on live equipment operating at 50 V and higher.

- Junction boxes: Are all the unused openings covered? See OSHA 1910.305(B), NFPA 400.8, and NEC 110.12(A). Are all live parts covered? See OSHA 1910.305(b)(2), NFPA 420.2, and NEC 314.25.

- Conductors: Is the overcurrent protection adequate for the conductor ampacity? See OSHA 1910.304(e), NFPA 410.9, and NEC 240.4.

R.E.C. safety practices

Safe work practices can be summed up in three words—recognize, evaluate, control (REC). Planning out a task, understanding code requirements, analyzing the power, equipment and working conditions, and then implementing safeguards to control risks and hazards are the essence of R.E.C.

Recognize hazards

The first step is to recognize and identify the existing and potential hazards associated with the work you need to perform. A task and hazard analysis and pre-job briefing are two of the tools you can utilize to ascertain the risks involved in your work for the day. It's a good idea to include everyone who will be involved in the task or associated work to discuss and plan for the hazards. Sometimes a coworker will think of hazards that you have overlooked, and it will ensure that everyone involved will be on the same page. Careful planning of safety procedures reduces the risk of injury. Determine whether everyone has been trained for the job they need to do that day. Do you need to present a safety training focused on specific risks that are present today? Decisions to lockout and tagout circuits and equipment and any other action plans should be made part of recognizing hazards. Here are some other topics to address:

- Is the existing wiring inadequate?

- Is there any potential for overloading circuits?

- Are there any exposed electrical parts?

- Will you be working around overhead power lines?

- Does any of the wiring have damaged insulation that will produce a shock?

- Are there any electrical systems or tools on the site that are not grounded or double insulated?

- Have you checked the condition of any power tools that will be used to confirm that they are not damaged and that all guards are in place?

- What PPE is required for the tasks to be performed?

- Have you reviewed the MSDS for any chemicals present on the site or that will be used that could be harmful?

- Will any work need to be performed from ladders or scaffolding and are these in good condition and set-up properly? Is there any chance of ladders coming in contact with energized circuits?

- Are the working conditions or equipment likely to be damp or wet or affected by humidity?

Evaluate the hazards

After you have identified all possible hazards, you can accurately evaluate the risk of injury from each hazard. Occasionally a risk may seem low or insignificant until you take the time to evaluate a hazard. One aspect of your day to consider is that job sites and conditions are constantly changing, and something what was not a problem yesterday could have evolved into a hazard today. It could be something as simple as the fact that it rained or snowed overnight and now equipment and site conditions are wet or slippery.

Combinations of hazards increase your risk. Improper grounding and a damaged tool greatly increase your risk. You will need to make decisions about the causes of any hazards in order to evaluate your risk. For example, if a GFCI keeps tripping while you are using a power tool, it is an indication that a problem exists. Don't just keep resetting the GFCI. Look for the reason the GFCI is tripping. Here are some typical examples of situations or conditions that require investigation and evaluation:

- Tripped circuit breakers and blown fuses: These indicate that too much current is flowing in a circuit or that a fault exists. This condition could be due to several factors, including faulty or damaged equipment or a short between conductors. You will need to isolate the cause in order to control the hazard.

- An electrical tool, appliance, wire, or connection feels warm to the touch: This may indicate that there is too much current in the circuit or equipment or that a fault exists. You will need to figure out which one of these potential factors is causing the problem.

■ A burning odor could be coming from overheated insulation. Worn, frayed, or damaged insulation around any wire or other conductor exposes the conductor, creating an electrical hazard. Damaged insulation could cause a short, leading to arcing or a fire, and contact with an exposed wire could cause a shock.

Controlling hazards

Once you have recognized and evaluated any electrical hazards, you have to control the risks to ensure your safety and the safety of the equipment and property you will be working on. Controlling hazards is accomplished by creating a safe work environment based on code-approved techniques and materials and by applying safe work practices.

A safe work environment reduces the chance of fires, burns, chemical hazards, falls, broken bones, and damaged equipment and materials. Safe work practices prevent electrical shocks, arcing, and hearing, back, head, and eye accidents and injuries that can last a lifetime. You can control many common hazards by identifying them in a timely manner, and even avoid them altogether with proper planning (Figure 12.10).

R.E.C. Process

Changing a Wall Ground Fault Circuit Interrupter (GFCI)

Task analysis	Hazard analysis	Hazard abatement
Removing the cover	Electric shock from exposed live wires	De-energize by opening circuit breaker or removing fuse
Removing old GFCI	Possible other live wires in opening	Test wires with appropriate voltmeter to ensure all wires are de-energized
Installing new GFCI	Possible connecting wires incorrectly	Check wiring diagrams to ensure proper connections
Replace cover and re-energize	Possible defective GFCI	Test GFCI

Figure 12.10   An REC example.

All of these precautions, plans, and practices would be easy to include in your day if a buzzer went off every time there was a hazard present. But you and I know that is not how it works. For most of us, there isn't someone standing behind us reminding us to put in our earplugs, or test for current, or not to open a panel because it's not de-energized. If you own your own business, you have to constantly try to balance profits with people's well-being. Maybe it would be easier if you made pillows for a living, but you are in the electrical trade. You work with and around one of the most dangerous elements in construction and you have to take the responsibility to protect yourself by working as safely as possible. Accidents are never planned, but safety can be. You owe it to yourself to take the little bit of extra time and effort required to ensure your safety everyday (Figure 12.00).

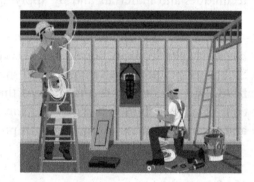

**STEPS TO CONTROLING
ELECTRICAL INCIDENTS**

- Treat all conductors, even those that have been de-energized, as if they are energized and dangerous.

- Verify that circuits are de-energized and test for any residual current before starting work.

- Lock out and tag out circuits and machines. Don't ever assume that the "other guy" has done this step. Always confirm lockout/tagout for yourself.

- Prevent overloaded wiring by using the right size and type of wire.

- Prevent exposure to live electrical parts by isolating them.

- Prevent shocking currents from electrical systems and tools by grounding them.

- Prevent shocking circuits by using GFCIs.

- Prevent too much current in circuits by using overcurrent protection devices.

- Prevent physical injuries by using Personal Protective Equipment that is matched to and rated for the work you need to perform. Take care of your PPE and replace old or damaged PPE to make sure that it will be effective.

Figure 12.00   Guide to Controlling Electrical Injuries.

Appendix

COMMON ELECTRICAL TERMS

General Terms

Adapter An accessory used for interconnecting non-mating devices or converting an existing device for modified use.

Ballast A transformer that steps down AC line voltage to voltage that can be used by fluorescent or other types of lighting. Ballast's may be electromagnetic or electronic

Cord Connector A portable receptacle designed for attachment to or provided with flexible cord, not intended for fixed mounting.

Flanged Inlet A plug intended for flush mounting on appliances or equipment to provide a means for power connection via a cord connector.

Flanged Outlet A receptacle intended for flush mounting on appliances or equipment to provide a means for power connection via an inserted plug.

Fluorescent Starter A device with a voltage-sensitive switch and a capacitor that provides a highvoltage pulse to start a fluorescent lamp. Rated in watts.

Lampholder A device with contacts that establishes mechanical and electrical connection to an inserted lamp.

Plug A device with male contacts intended for insertion into a receptacle to establish electrical connection between the attached flexible cord and the conductors connected to the receptacle.

Receptacle A device with female contacts designed for fixed installation in a structure or piece of equipment and which is intended to establish electrical connection with an inserted plug.

Switch A device for making, breaking, or changing the connections in an electric circuit.

Wallplate A plate designed to enclose an electrical box, with or without a device installed within the box.

Cord Connectors

Angle A connector that allows the attached flexible cord to exit at right angles.

Corrosion Resistant A connector constructed of special materials and/or suitably plated metal parts that is designed to withstand corrosive environments. Corrosion resistant devices must pass the ASTM B117-13 five-hundred hour Salt Spray (Fog) Test with no visible corrosion.

Dust Proof A connector designed so that dust will not interfere with its operation. The IP Suitability Rating designates the degree of protection a device offers against the ingress of foreign objects (e.g. IP 20).

Explosion Proof A connector constructed to meet the requirements of hazardous locations as defined by the National Electrical Code, NFPA-70.

Hospital Grade A connector designed to meet the performance requirements of high-abuse areas typically found in health care facilities. These connectors are tested to the Hospital Grade requirements of Underwriters Laboratories Inc. Standard 498.

Locking A connector designed to lock an inserted plug with a matching blade configuration when the plug is rotated in a clockwise direction. The plug can only be removed by first turning it in a counter-clockwise direction.

Midget A connector designed with a smaller body diameter than standard connectors with a similar rating.

Pin and Sleeve A connector with hollow, cylindrical sleeve-type contacts.

Straight Blade A non-locking connector into which mating plugs are inserted at a right angle to the plane of the connector face.

Weatherproof A connector specially constructed so that exposure to weather will not interfere with its operation.

Adapter Variations

<u>Cube Tap</u> An adapter that converts one receptacle opening into multiple openings.

<u>Current Tap</u> An adapter designed for medium base lampholders which has one or two receptacle openings. Available with or without integral switch.

<u>Duplex</u> An adapter that provides two female receptacle openings when plugged into a single receptacle opening.

<u>Grounding</u> An adapter that converts a two-wire receptacle opening into a two-pole, three-wire grounding receptacle opening.

<u>Lampholder</u> A threaded adapter that converts the thread size of the lampholder in which it is inserted so that the lampholder can accept an incandescent lamp bulb of a different size thread.

<u>Molded-On</u> An adapter that is factory molded to a length of flexible cord.

<u>Series</u> An adapter wired in series to a flexible cord containing an in-line switch used to control electrical equipment plugged into the adapter.

<u>"Y" Type</u> An adapter in the form of a letter "Y", having two cord connectors on one end and a male plug on the other end.

<u>"W" Type</u> Same as "Y" type, except having three cord connectors arranged in the form of the letter "W".

Lampholders

Bayonet Designed for incandescent lamps having an unthreaded metal shell with two diametrically opposite keyways that mate with the keyways on the lampholder. Pushing down on the bulb and turning it clockwise in the lampholder locks the bulb in place.

Candelabra A small screw-base threaded lampholder designed for candelabra-base incandescent lamps commonly used in chandeliers, night lights, and ornamental lighting.

Circline A four-contact, double-ended lampholder designed for use with tubular, circular fluorescent lamps.

Compact Fluorescent A lampholder designed for the Compact Fluorescent Lamps (CFL's) that are increasingly being used to replace incandescent lamps for energy efficiency.

Dimmer An electronic device with either a round knob, slide lever or finger-tip controlled buttons used to dim/brighten incandescent lighting. Available in a variety of wattages; fluorescent version also available.

Double-Contact Recessed Designed for high-output fluorescent lamps.

Edison Base An internally-threaded lampholder, with the inner shell approx. 1" in diameter. Designed for widely-used standard medium base lamps.

Electrolier Similar to the Edison Medium Base lampholder, but with a smaller outer diameter. Incandescent Designed for use with all manufactured incandescent lamps, most of which have threaded bases.

Key A lampholder with a flat or round "key" knob that operates an internal switching mechanism ("Keyless" lampholders do not provide an internal switching mechanism).

Lumiline A specially designed lampholder for tubular Lumiline-type incandescent lamps, typically used in bathrooms and retail display cases.

Mogul The largest screw-in type lampholder, designed for mogul incandescent lamps with a screw base of approx. 11/2" dia. Used in street lights and numerous commercial/industrial applications. Medium Bi-Pin A fluorescent lampholder with two contacts, used in pairs. For type T-8 tubular fluorescent lamps, approx. 1" in diameter.

Miniature Bi-Pin Similar to medium bi-pin lampholders, but designed for type T-5 tubular fluorescent lamps, approx. 5/8" in diameter.

Outlet Box Medium-base incandescent lampholder designed for mounting in 31/4" or 4" electrical boxes. Available with or without pull-chain mechanism, and with or without built-in receptacle. Pull-Chain An incandescent lampholder with an internal switching mechanism that is activated by pulling down on a beaded chain or cord.

Push-Through An incandescent lampholder with an insulated lever that is pushed from either side to activate an internal ON/OFF switching mechanism.

Slimline Single-Pin A fluorescent lampholder with a single contact designed for Slimline fluorescent lamps such as the T-12 (11/2" dia.), T-8 (1" dia.), and the smaller version T-6 (3/4" dia.).

Snap-In An incandescent or compact fluorescent lampholder with factory-assembled spring clips that securely snap into a panel cutout without requiring additional fasteners. Surface-Mounted A lampholder of any type that mounts on a flat or plane surface.

Receptacles

AL/CU 30A, 50A or 60A receptacles designated for use with aluminum or copper circuit conductors, identified by "AL/CU" stamped on the device. Receptacles without this designation must never be used with aluminum circuit conductors.

Clock Hanger A single, recessed receptacle with a specialized cover plate that provides a hook or other means of supporting a wall clock.

CO/ALR 15A or 20A receptacles designated for use with aluminum or copper circuit conductors, identified by "CO/ALR" stamped on the device. Receptacles without this designation must never be used with aluminum circuit conductors.

Corrosion Resistant A receptacle constructed of special materials and/or suitably plated metal parts that is designed to withstand corrosive environments. Corrosion resistant devices must pass the ASTM B117-13 five-hundred hour Salt Spray (Fog) Test with no visible corrosion.

Display Receptacle with a special cover plate intended for flush mounting on raised floors or walls.

Duplex Two receptacles built with a common body and mounting means; accepts two plugs.

Explosion Proof A receptacle constructed to meet the requirements of hazardous locations as defined by the National Electrical Code, NFPA-70.

Four-In-One or "Quad" A receptacle in a common housing that accepts up to four plugs. Four-In-One receptacles can be installed in place of duplex receptacles mounted in a single-gang box, providing a convenient means of adding receptacles without rewiring.

GFCI (Ground Fault Circuit Interrupter) A receptacle with a built in circuit that will detect leakage current to ground on the load side of the device. When the GFCI detects leakage current to ground, it will interrupt power to the load side of the device, preventing a hazardous ground fault condition. GFCI receptacles must conform to UL Standard 943 Class A requirements, and their use is required by the National Electric Code NFPA-70 in a variety of indoor and outdoor locations.

Hospital Grade A receptacle designed to meet the performance requirements of high-abuse areas typically found in health care facilities. These receptacles are tested to the Hospital Grade requirements of Underwriters Laboratories Inc. Standard 498.

Interchangeable A receptacle or combination of receptacles with a common mounting dimension that may be installed on a single or multiple-opening mounting strap.

Isolated Ground Receptacles intended for use in an Isolated Grounding system where the ground path is isolated from the facility grounding system. The grounding connection on these receptacles is isolated from the mounting strap.

Lighted (Illuminated) A receptacle with a face that becomes illuminated when the device is connected to an energized electrical circuit.

Locking A receptacle designed to lock an inserted plug with a matching blade configuration when the plug is rotated in a clockwise direction. The plug can only be removed by first turning it in a counter-clockwise direction.

Safety or Tamper-Resistant A receptacle specially constructed so that access to its energized contacts is limited. Tamper-resistant receptacles are required by the National Electric Code NFPA-70 in specific pediatric care areas in health care facilities.

Single A receptacle that accepts only one plug.

Split-Circuit A duplex receptacle that allows each receptacle to be wired to separate circuits. Most duplex receptacles provide break-off tabs that allow them to be converted into split-circuit receptacles.

Straight Blade A non-locking receptacle into which mating plugs are inserted at a right angle to the plane of the receptacle face.

Surface-Mounted Any receptacle that mounts on a flat or plane surface.

Surge-Suppression A receptacle with built-in circuitry designed to protect its load side from high-voltage transients and surges. The circuitry will limit transient voltage peaks to help protect sensitive electronic equipment such as PC's, modems, audio/video equipment, etc.

Triplex A receptacle with a common mounting means which accepts three plugs.

Weatherproof A receptacle specially constructed so that exposure to weather will not interfere with its operation.

Surge Suppression

Clamping Voltage The peak voltage that can be measured after a Surge Protective Device has limited or "clamped" a transient voltage surge. Clamping voltage must be determined by using IEEE Standard C62 testing and evaluated by UL Standard 1449.

Joule Rating The measurement of a Surge Protective Device's ability to absorb heat energy created by transient surges. Note that the Joule rating is not a part of IEEE or UL Standards. It is not as significant a specification as Clamping Voltage, Maximum Surge Current and other parameters recognized by these agencies.

Transient Voltage Surges High-speed, high-energy electrical disturbances present on AC power lines and data and communication lines, generated by utility switching, motor-load switching and lightning strikes.

Response Time The interval of time it takes for a surge protective device to react to a transient voltage surge. Note that this parameter is not a part of IEEE or UL Standards and is only based on estimations made by manufacturers.

Surge Protective Device See "Transient Voltage Surge Suppressor (TVSS)" definition. Transient Voltage Surge Suppressor (TVSS) A device designed to protect sensitive electronic equipment such as computers and computer peripherals, logic controls, audio/video equipment and a wide range of microprocessor-based (computer chip) equipment from the harmful effects of transient voltage surges. Also referred to as a Surge Protective Device (SPD).

Maximum (Peak) Surge Current The peak surge current a Surge Protective Device can withstand, based on IEEE Standard C62.45 test waveforms.

MOV (Metal Oxide Varistor) The primary component used in most Surge Protective Devices to clamp down transient voltages.

UL 1449 Listing The industry standard for Surge Protective Devices. A Surge Protective Device must have a UL 1449 Surge Suppression rating on its label in order to verify that the device has been tested with IEEE standardized waveforms. Devices without this identification should not be considered reliable surge protective devices.

Wallplates

Combination A multiple- gang wallplate with openings in each gang to accommodate different devices.

Flush A wallplate designed for flush-mounting with wall surfaces or the plane surfaces of electrical equipment.

Gang A term that describes the number of devices a wallplate is sized to fit (i.e. "2- gang" designates two devices).

Midway Wallplates that are approx. 3/8" higher and wider than the standard size that can be mounted onto larger volume outlet boxes and/or used to hide wall surface irregularities. These wallplates are approx. 1/4" deep to ensure a proper fit when used with protruding devices.
Oversized Wallplates that are approx. 3/4" higher and wider than the standard size and are used to conceal greater wall irregularities than those hidden by Midway wallplates. These wallplates are approx. 1/4" deep to ensure a proper fit when used with protruding devices.

Modular Individual-section wallplates with different openings that can be configured into a multigang plate.

Multi-Gang A wallplate that has two or more gangs.

Tandem A wallplate with individual gangs arranged vertically one above the other.

Weatherproof (with Cover Closed) A UL Listed cover that meets specific test standards for use in wet and damp locations with the cover closed.

Weatherproof (with Cover Open) A UL Listed cover that meets specific test standards for use in wet and damp locations with the cover open or closed.

Switches

<u>AC/DC</u> A switch designated for use with either Alternating Current (AC) or Direct Current (DC).

<u>AC Only</u> A switch designated for use with Alternating Current (AC) only.

<u>Dimmer</u> A switch with electronic circuitry that provides DIM/BRIGHT control of lighting loads.
Door A momentary contact switch, usually installed on a doorjamb, that is activated when the door is opened or closed.

<u>Double-Pole, Single-Throw (DPST)</u> A switch that makes or breaks the connection of two circuit conductors in a single branch circuit. This switch has four terminal screws and ON/OFF markings.

<u>Double-Pole, Double-Throw (DPDT)</u> A switch that makes or breaks the connection of two conductors to two separate circuits. This switch has six terminal screws and is available in both momentary and maintained contact versions, and may also have a center OFF position.

<u>Feed-Through</u> An in-line switch that can be attached at any point on a length of flexible cord to provide switching control of attached equipment.

<u>Flush-Mounted</u> A switch designed for flush installation with the surface of a panel or equipment.
Four-Way A switch used in conjunction with two 3-Way switches to control a single load (such as a light fixture) from three or more locations. This switch has four terminal screws and no ON/OFF marking.

<u>Horsepower Rated</u> A switch with a marked horsepower rating, intended for use in switching motor loads.

<u>Interchangeable</u> A switch or combination of switches with a common mounting dimension that may be installed on a single or multiple-opening mounting strap.

Lighted Handle A switch with an integral lamp in its actuator (toggle, rocker or pushbutton) that illuminates when the switch is connected to an energized circuit and the actuator is in the OFF position.

Low-Voltage A switch rated for use on low-voltage circuits of 50 volts or less.

L-Rated A switch specially designated with the letter "L" in its rating that is rated for controlling tungsten filament lamps on AC circuits only.

Maintained Contact A switch where the actuator (toggle, rocker, pushbutton or key mechanism) makes and retains circuit contact when moved to the ON position. The contacts will only be opened when the actuator is manually moved to the OFF position. Ordinary light switches are maintained contact switches.

Manual Motor Controller A switch designed for controlling small DC or AC motor loads, without overload protection.

Mercury A type of switch that uses mercury as the contact means for making and breaking an electrical circuit.

Momentary Contact A switch that makes circuit contact only as long as the actuator (toggle, rocker, pushbutton or key mechanism) is held in the ON position, after which it returns automatically to the OFF position. This is a "Normally Open" switch. A "Normally Closed" switch will break circuit contact as long as it is held in the OFF position, and then automatically return to the ON position. Available in "Center OFF" versions with both Momentary ON and Momentary OFF positions.

Pendant A type of switch designed for installation at the end of a length of portable cord or cable.

Pilot Light A switch with an integral lamp in its actuator (toggle, rocker or pushbutton) that illuminates when the switch is connected to an energized circuit and the actuator is in the ON position.

<u>Pull</u> A switch where the making or breaking of contacts is controlled by pulling downward or outward on the actuator mechanism.

<u>Push Button</u> A switch with an actuator mechanism that is operated by depressing a button.

<u>Rotary</u> A switch where rotating the actuator in a clockwise direction makes the circuit connection, and then rotating the actuator in either the same or opposite direction breaks the connection.

<u>Single-Pole, Double-Throw (SPDT)</u> A switch that makes or breaks the connection of a single conductor with either of two other single conductors. This switch has 3 terminal screws, and is commonly used in pairs and called a "Three-Way" switch.

<u>Single-Pole, Single-Throw (SPST)</u> A switch that makes or breaks the connection of a single conductor in a single branch circuit. This switch has two screw terminals and ON/OFF designations. It is commonly referred to as a "Single-Pole" Switch.

<u>Slide</u> A switch with a slide-action actuator for making or breaking circuit contact. Dimmer switches and fan speed controls are also available with slide-action mechanisms for lighting and fan speed control.

<u>Surface-Mounted</u> Any switch that mounts on a flat or plane surface.

<u>Three-Position, Center OFF</u> A two circuit switch, either maintained or momentary contact, where the OFF position is designated as the center position of the actuator.

<u>Three-Way</u> A switch, always used in pairs, that controls a single load such as a light fixture from two locations. This switch has three terminal screws and has no ON/OFF marking.

<u>Time Delay</u> A switch with an integral mechanism or electronic circuit that will automatically switch a load OFF at a predetermined time interval.

<u>Timer</u> A switch with an integral mechanism or electronic circuit that can be set to switch an electrical load ON at a predetermined time.

<u>Toggle</u> A switch with a lever-type actuator that makes or breaks switch contact as its position is changed.

<u>T-Rated</u> A switch specially designated with the letter "T" in its rating that is rated for controlling tungsten filament lamps on direct current (DC) or alternating current (AC) circuits.

BASIC ELECTRICAL THEORY

Series Direct Current Circuits

◆ Total Resistance of a series circuit is equal to the sum of the individual resistances.

◆ The same current flows through each part of a series circuit.

◆ The total voltage across a series circuit is equal to the sum of the individual voltage drops.

◆ The voltage drop across a resistor in a series circuit is proportionate to the size of the resistor.

◆ The total power dissipated in a series circuit is equal to the sum of the individual power dissapation

Parallel Direct Current Circuits

The same voltage is present across each branch of a parallel circuit and is equal to the source voltage.

Current that flows through a branch of a parallel network is inversely proportional to the amount of resistance of the branch.

The total power loss in a parallel circuit is equal to the sum of the individual power dissapation.

The total current of a parallel circuit is equal to the sum of the currents of the individual branches of the circuit.

The total resistance of a parallel circuit is equal to the shared sum of the reciprocals of the individual resistances of the circuit.

PARALLEL CIRCUIT RULES

$$\text{TOTAL VOLTAGE} = E(1) = E(2) = E(3)$$

$$\text{TOTAL RESISTANCE} = \frac{\text{VOLTS}}{\text{AMPERES}}$$

$$\text{VOLTS} = \frac{\text{TOTAL VOLTAGE}}{\text{TOTAL AMPERES}}$$

TO DETERMINE THE TOTAL RESISTANCE IN A PARALLEL CIRCUIT WHEN THE TOTAL CURRENT AND TOTAL VOLTAGE ARE UNKNOWN USE EITHER OF THE FOLLOWING FORMULAS:

$$RT = \frac{1}{\dfrac{1}{R1} + \dfrac{1}{R2} + \dfrac{1}{R3} + \ldots\ldots \text{etc}}$$

FOR TWO RESISTORS IN PARALLEL USE THIS FORMULA CALLED THE "PRODUCT OVER THE SUM"

$$RT = \frac{R(1) * R(2)}{R(1) + R(2)}$$

**POWER IN SINGLE PHASE RESISTIVE CIRCUITS
WITH A POWER FACTOR OF 100 PERCENT**

◆ To determine the power used by an individual resistor in a
SERIES CIRCUIT USE THE FOLLOWING FORMULA:

$$\textbf{POWER} = \textbf{I}^2 \times \textbf{R}$$

◆ To determine the power used by an individual resistor in a
PARALLEL CIRCUIT USE THIS FORMULA:

$$\textbf{POWER} = \frac{\textbf{E}^2}{\textbf{R}}$$

◆ To determine the total power used by an INDIVIDUAL
CIRCUIT USE THIS FORMULA:

POWER = E (TOTAL VOLTAGE) × I (TOTAL CURRENT)

**POWER IN ALTERNATING CURRENT CIRCUITS WHERE
POWER FACTOR IS NOT 100 PERCENT**

POWER = E × I × POWER FACTOR (FOR SINGLE PHASE)

**POWER = E × I × 1.732 X POWER FACTOR (FOR THREE
PHASE)**

VOLT-AMPERES = E × I (FOR SINGLE PHASE)

VOLT-AMPERES = E × I × 1.732 (FOR THREE PHASE)

$$\textbf{POWER FACTOR} = \frac{\textbf{TRUE POWER}}{\textbf{APPARENT POWER}}$$

**POWER CALCULATED IN THIS WAY IS CALLED <u>TRUE
POWER</u> OR <u>REAL POWER</u>**

**<u>APPARENT POWER</u> FOUND BY CALCULATING VOLT-
AMPERES.**

MOTOR APPLICATION FORMULAS

$$\frac{\text{HORSEPOWER}}{\text{(for three phase motors)}} = \frac{1.732 \times \text{VOLTS} \times \text{AMPERES} \times \text{EFFICIENCY} \times \text{power factor}}{746}$$

$$\frac{\text{THREE PHASE AMPERES}}{\text{(for three phase motors)}} = \frac{746 \times \text{HORSEPOWER}}{1.732 \times \text{VOLTS} \times \text{EFFICIENCY} \times \text{POWER FACTOR}}$$

$$\text{SYNCHRONOUS RPM} = \frac{\text{HERTZ} \times 120}{\text{NUMBER OF POLES}}$$

	Maximum Horsepower for NEMA-Rated Motor Starters			
	Single-Phase		Three-Phase	
NEMA Size	115 Volt	230 Volt	208/230 Volt	460/575 Volt
00	1/3	1	1.5	2
0	1	2	3	5
1	2	3	7.5	10
2	3	7.5	10/15	25
3			25/30	50
4			40/50	100
5			75/100	200

GENERAL ELECTRICAL THEORY

⚡ THE TOTAL RESISTANCE OF RESISTORS RUN IN PARALLEL IS ALWAYS <u>LESS THAN</u> THE VALUE OF ANY ONE RESISTOR.

⚡ THE TOTAL RESISTANCE OF PARALLEL RESISTORS THAT ARE ALL THE SAME VALUE IS THE VALUE ÷ BY THE NUMBER OF RESISTORS.

⚡ POWER FACTOR MEASURES HOW FAR CURRENT LEADS OR LAGS A VOLTAGE.

⚡ 746 WATTS IS EQUAL TO ONE HORSEPOWER

⚡ EFFICIENCY IS EQUAL TO OUTPUT DIVIDED BY INPUT

⚡ IN INDUCTIVE CIRCUITS CURRENT LAGS VOLTAGE.

⚡ IN CAPACITIVE CIRCUITS CURRENT LEADS VOLTAGE

ELECTRICAL FORMULAS

◆ <u>**Electrical Formulas Based on 60 Hz**</u>

Effective (RMS) AC Amperes = Peak Amperes × 0.707

Effective (RMS) AC Volts = Peak Volts × 0.707

Efficiency = Output/Input

Horsepower = Output Watts/746

Input = Output/Efficiency

Neutral Current (Wye) = $\sqrt{A^2 + B^2 + C^2 - (AB + BC + AC)}$

Output = Input × Efficiency

Peak AC Volts = Effective (RMS) AC Volts × $\sqrt{2}$

Peak Amperes = Effective (RMS) Amperes × $\sqrt{2}$

Power Factor (PF) = Watts/VA

VA (apparent power) = Volts × Ampere or Watts/Power Factor

VA 1-Phase = Volts × Amperes

VA 3-Phase = Volts × Amperes × $\sqrt{3}$

Watts - Single-Phase = Volts × Amperes × Power Factor

Watts - Three-Phase = Volts × Amperes × Power Factor × $\sqrt{3}$

<u>OHM'S LAW</u>

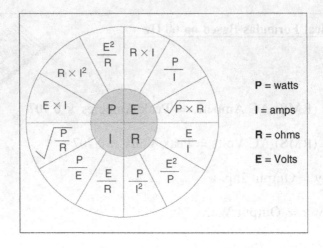

P = watts

I = amps

R = ohms

E = Volts

ELECTRICAL CONVERSIONS

Busbar Ampacity AL = 700A Sq. in. and
CU = 1000A Sq. in.

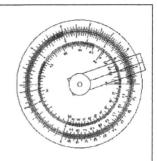

Centimeters = Inches × 2.54

Inch = 0.0254 Meters

Inch = 2.54 Centimeters

Inch = 25.4 Millimeters

Kilometer = 0.6213 Miles

Length of Coiled Wire = Diameter of Coil (average) × Number of
Coils × π

Meter = 39.37 Inches

Millimeter = 0.03937 Inch

Temp C = (Temp F − 32)/1.8

Temp F = (Temp C × 1.8) + 32

Yard = 0.9144 Meters

CURRENT FORMULAS

◆ **Parallel Circuits**

~ Total resistance is always less than the smallest resistor

$$RT = 1/(1/R1 + 1/R2 + 1/R3 \text{ (etc)}$$

~ Total current is equal to the sum of the currents of all parallel resistors

~ Total power is equal to the sum of power of all parallel resistors

~ Voltage is the same across each of the parallel resistors

◆ **Series Circuits**

~ Total resistance is equal to the sum of all the resistors

~ Current in the circuit remains the same through all the resistors

~ Voltage source is equal to the sum of voltage drops of all resistors

~ Power of the circuit is equal to the sum of the power of all resistors

◆ **Voltage Drop**

VD (1-Phase) = 2KID/CM

VD (3-Phase) = $\sqrt{3}$ KID/CM

CM (1-Phase) = 2KID/VD

CM (3-Phase) = $\sqrt{3}$ KID/VD

ARC FAULT CURRENTS

Bolted Fault Current	Arc Fault Current
@ 480 V	
10 kA	= 6.56 kA
20 kA	= 11.85 kA
30 kA	= 16.76 kA
40 kA	= 21.43 kA

STANDARD VOLTAGES

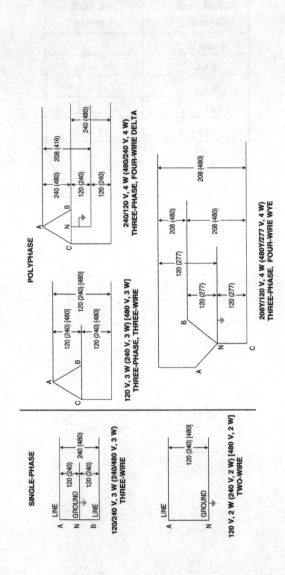

VOLTAGE DROP INFORMATION

VOLTAGE DROP

Voltage is contained in a short conductor because the power flow meets less resistance

Voltage spreads out in a longer conductor and the resistance to the power flow increases and the voltage drops

◆Voltage Drop Formulas

Single Phase (2 or 3 wire)	VD =	$\dfrac{2 \times K \times I \times L}{CM}$	**K** = ohms per mil foot **(Copper = 12.9 at 75°)** **(Alum = 21.2 at 75°)** *Note: K value changes with temperature. See NEC Chapter 9, Table 8* **L** = Length of conductor in feet **I** = Current in conductor (amperes) **CM** = Circular mil area of conductor

<u>TRANSFORMER CALCULATIONS</u>

Secondary Amperes 1-Phase = VA/Volts

Secondary Amperes 3-Phase = VA/Volts $\times \sqrt{3}$

Secondary Available Fault 1-Phase = VA/(Volts $\times$ %impedance)

Secondary Available Fault 3-Phase = VA/(Volts $\times \sqrt{3} \times$ % Impedance)

Delta 4-Wire: Line Amperes = Phase (one winding) Amperes $\times \sqrt{3}$

Delta 4-Wire: Line Volts = Phase (one Winding) Volts

Delta 4-Wire: High-Leg Voltage (L-to-G) = Phase (one winding) Volts $\times$ 0.5 $\times \sqrt{3}$

Wye: Line Volts = Phase (one winding) Volts $\times \sqrt{3}$

Wye: Line Amperes = Phase (one winding) Amperes

NEC QUICK CODE REFERENCE GUIDE

AC-DC: Panelboards & Ratings -
SECTION [408.36 (C)

Air Conditioners & Refrigeration
Equipment - Article 440

Appliances: Load Calculations - SECTION [220.14], [220.40]
Table [220.55]

Audio Signal Processing: Grounding - SECTION [640.7]

Bathroom Wiring: Branch Circuits -SECTION [210.11 (C) (3);
Receptacles SECTION [210.8 (A)(1)

Branch Circuits: Articles 210 & 220

Breakers and Fuse Ratings: SECTION [240.6(A)]

Conductor Ampacity: SECTION [310.15] and Table [310.16]

Conductors: Number (quantity) Allowed - Chapter 9,
Table 1 - Annex C

Equipment Grounding Conductors: SECTION [250.122]

Grounding Electrode Conductors: SECTION [250.66]

Motor Conductor Sizing: SECTION [430.22] for Single and
SECTION [430.24] for Multiple

Feeders: Calculation of loads - SECTION [215.2(A), [220.40]

Fire Alarm Systems: Conductors: SECTION [760.27]

Flexible Metal Conduit: Number of Conductors: SECTION [348.22]

Generators: Article 445

Hazardous Locations: Article 500

Loads: Calculations: Article 220, Annex D

Motor Short-Circuit Protection: SECTION [430.52]

Panelboards: Distribution - SECTIONS 550, 551, 552

Service Entrance Conductors: Article 230

Transformer Overcurrent Protection: SECTION [450.3]

◆**Voltage and Current:**

Primary (p) secondary (s) Power(p) = power (s) or $E_p \times I_p = E_s \times I_s$

•Ep =	$\dfrac{Es \times Is}{Ip}$
•Ip =	$\dfrac{Es \times Is}{Ep}$
•Is =	$\dfrac{Ep \times Ip}{Es}$
•Es =	$\dfrac{Ep \times Ip}{Is}$

Voltage and Turns in Coil:

Voltage (p) × Turns (s) = Voltage (s) × Turns (p) or $E_p \times T_s = E_s \times I_p$

•Ep =	$\dfrac{Es \times Ip}{Ts}$
•Ts =	$\dfrac{Es \times Tp}{Ep}$
•Tp =	$\dfrac{Ep \times Ts}{Es}$
•Es =	$\dfrac{Ep \times Ts}{Tp}$

◆ AC/DC Formulas

E = Voltage / I = Amps /W = Watts / PF = Power Factor / Eff = Efficiency / HP = Horsepower

To Find	Direct Current	AC / 1phase 115v or 120v	AC / 1phase 208,230, or 240v	AC 3 phase All Voltages
Amps when Horsepower is Known	$\dfrac{HP \times 746}{E \times Eff}$	$\dfrac{HP \times 746}{E \times Eff \times PF}$	$\dfrac{HP \times 746}{E \times Eff \times PF}$	$\dfrac{HP \times 746}{1.73 \times E \times Eff \times PF}$
Amps when Kilowatts is known	$\dfrac{kW \times 1000}{E}$	$\dfrac{kW \times 1000}{E \times PF}$	$\dfrac{kW \times 1000}{E \times PF}$	$\dfrac{kW \times 1000}{1.73 \times E \times PF}$
Amps when kVA is known		$\dfrac{kVA \times 1000}{E}$	$\dfrac{kVA \times 1000}{E}$	$\dfrac{kVA \times 1000}{1.73 \times E}$
Kilowatts	$\dfrac{I \times E}{1000}$	$\dfrac{I \times E \times PF}{1000}$	$\dfrac{I \times E \times PF}{1000}$	$\dfrac{I \times E \times 1.73\, PF}{1000}$
Kilovolt-Amps		$\dfrac{I \times E}{1000}$	$\dfrac{I \times E}{1000}$	$\dfrac{I \times E \times 1.73}{1000}$
Horsepower (output)	$\dfrac{I \times E \times Eff}{746}$	$\dfrac{I \times E \times Eff \times PF}{746}$	$\dfrac{I \times E \times Eff \times PF}{746}$	$\dfrac{I \times E \times Eff \times 1.73 \times PF}{746}$

◆ Power - DC Circuits

Watts = E xI
Amps = W / E

◆ AC Efficiency and Power Factor Formulas

E = Voltage / I = Amps /W = Watts / PF = Power Factor / Eff = Efficiency / HP = Horsepower

To Find:	Single Phase	Three Phase
Efficiency	$\dfrac{746 \times HP}{E \times I \times PF}$	$\dfrac{746 \times HP}{E \times I \times PF \times 1.732}$
Power Factor	$\dfrac{Input\ Watts}{V \times A}$	$\dfrac{Input\ Watts}{E \times I \times 1.732}$

NEC MINIMUM CONDUCTOR SIZES

CONDUCTOR VOLTAGE	Copper	Aluminum or Copper-Clad Aluminum
0 - 2000 VOLTS	#14 AWG	#12 AWG
2100 - 4000 VOLTS 4001 - 8000 VOLTS	#8 AWG	#8 AWG
8001 - 10,000 VOLTS 10,001 - 15,000 VOLTS	#2 AWG	#2 AWG
15,001 - 25,000 VOLTS 25,001 - 28,000 VOLTS	#1 AWG	#1 AWG
28,001 - 35,000 VOLTS	1/0 AWG	1/0 AWG

STANDARD NEC CABLE SIZES

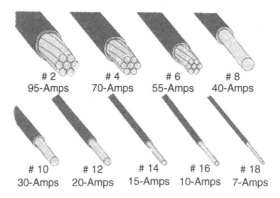

| # 2 | # 4 | # 6 | # 8 |
| 95-Amps | 70-Amps | 55-Amps | 40-Amps |

| # 10 | # 12 | # 14 | # 16 | # 18 |
| 30-Amps | 20-Amps | 15-Amps | 10-Amps | 7-Amps |

METRIC EQUIVALENT CHART

Matric conversion

Linear Measure

1 centimeter	0.3937 inch
1 inch	2.54 centimeters
1 decimeter	3.937 in., 0.328 foot
1 foot	3.048 decimeters
1 meter	39.37 inches, 1.0936 yds.
1 yard	0.9144 meter
1 dekameter	1.9884 rods
1 rod	0.5029 dekameter
1 kilometer	0.62137 mile
1 mile	1.6094 kilometers

Square Measure

1 sq. centimeter	0.1550 sq. inches
1 sq. inch	6.452 sq. centimeters
1 sq. decimeter	0.1076 sq. foot
1 sq. foot	9.2903 sq. decimeters
1 sq. meter	1.196 yards
1 sq. yard	0.8361 sq. meter
1 hectare	2.471 acres
1 acre	0.4047 hectare
1 sq. kilometer	0.386 sq. mile

Measure of Volume

1 cu. centimeter	0.06 1 cu. inch
1 cu. Inch	16.39 cu. centimeters
1 cu. decimeter	0.0353 cu. foot
1 cu. foot	28.3 17 cu. decimeters
1 cu. yard	0.7646 cu. meters
1 cu. meter	0.2759 cord
1 cord	3.625 steres
1 liter	0.908 qt. dry 1.0567 qts. liq.
1 quart dry	1.101 liters
1 quart liquid	0.9463 liter
1 dekaliter	2.6417 gals, 1.135 pks.
1 gallon	0.3785 dekaliter
1 peck	0.881 dekaliter
1 hectoliter	2.8378 bushels
1 bushel	0.3524 hectoliter

Weights

1 gram	0.03527 ounce
1 ounce	28.35 grams
1 kilogram	2.2046 pounds
1 pound	0.4536 kilogram

INCH TO MM CHART

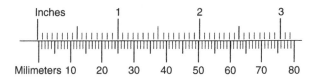

Use the tool above to convert Inches to Milimeters
Example 1/2 inch = 12mm "Milimeters"

GROUNDING DIAGRAM

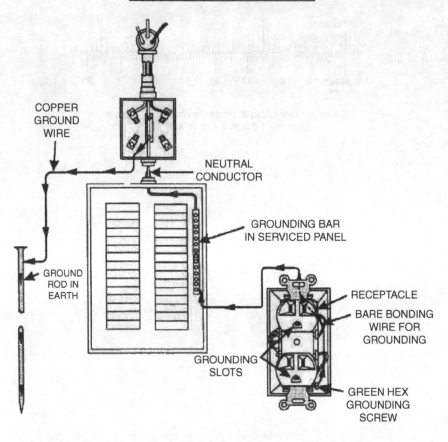

COPPER GROUND WIRE

NEUTRAL CONDUCTOR

GROUNDING BAR IN SERVICED PANEL

GROUND ROD IN EARTH

RECEPTACLE

BARE BONDING WIRE FOR GROUNDING

GROUNDING SLOTS

GREEN HEX GROUNDING SCREW

FIRE EXTINGUISHER SYMBOLS

 ORDINARY COMBUSTIBLES

Think ASHES: paper, wood, cardboard

 FLAMMABLE LIQUIDS

Think BARREL: flammable liquids (cylinders)

 ELECTRICAL EQUIPMENT

Think CIRCUITS: electrical fires

TYPICAL ARC FLASH LABEL

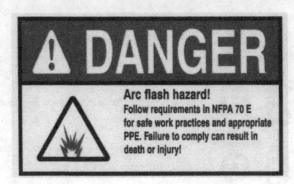

OSHA COLOR CODES

Color	Message	Sample Applications
White/Black	Designates traffic and housekeeping markings.	Boundaries of traffic isles, stairways, and directional signs.
Orange	Designates "warning" and dangerous parts of machinery or energized equipment which could cause injury.	Background color for WARNING safety signs, labels, and tags. Marking hazardous parts of machines with may cut, crush, or otherwise injure. Emphasizing hazards when enclosure doors are open or when gear, belt, or other guards around moving equipment are opened or removed, exposing unguarded hazards. Marking exposed edges of pulleys, gears, rollers, cutting devices, power jaws, etc.
Blue	Warning against starting or moving equipment under repairs.	Ladders, scaffolding, electrical controls, elevator starting controls, and other machinery.
Red	Designates "danger," "stop" and location of fire protection equipment and apparatus.	Emergency stop buttons, bars, and electrical switches. Safety cans or other portable containers of flammable liquids. Fire alarm boxes, fire extinguishers, fire hydrants.
Purple	Designates radiation hazards.	Rooms with X-ray equipment in use
Green	Designates "safety" and location of first aid equipment.	Background color for general safety signs including gas masks, first aid kits, stretchers, safety deluge showers, safety bulletin boards, and emergency exit routes.
Yellow	Designates "caution" for marking physical hazards such as: striking against, stumbling, falling, tripping, and "caught in between."	Background color for CAUTION safety signs, labels, and tags. Low beams, conveyors, doorway projections, and hand rails. Storage cabinets for flammable materials. For containers of flammable or combustible materials. Containers for corrosive, or unstable materials.

OSHA OFFICES

◆**Region 1**

Regional Office
JFK Federal Building, Room E340
Boston, Massachusetts 02203
(617) 565-9860
(617) 565-9827 FAX

Area Offices
Connecticut | Massachusetts | Maine | New Hampshire | Rhode Island |
Vermont

Bridgeport Area Office
Clark Building
1057 Broad Street, 4th Floor
Bridgeport, Connecticut 06604
(203) 579-5581
Fax: (203) 579-5516

Hartford Area Office
Federal Building
450 Main Street, Room 613
Hartford, Connecticut 06103
(860) 240-3152
Fax: (860) 240-3155

North Boston Area Office
Shattuck Office Center
138 River Road, Suite 102
Andover, MA 01810
(978)837-4460
Fax: 978-837-4455

South Boston Area Office
639 Granite Street, 4th Floor
Braintree, Massachusetts 02184
(617) 565-6924
Fax: (617) 565-6923

Springfield Area Office
1441 Main Street, Room 550
Springfield, Massachusetts 01103-1493
(413) 785-0123
Fax: (413) 785-0136

Bangor District Office
382 Harlow Street
Bangor, ME 04401
(207) 941-8177
Fax: (207) 941-8179

Augusta Area Office
E.S. Muskie Federal Bldg
40 Western Ave., Room G-26
Augusta, ME 04330
(207) 626-9160
Fax: (207) 622-8213

Concord Area Office
J.C. Cleveland Federal Bldg
53 Pleasant Street, Room 3901
Concord, New Hampshire 03301
(603) 225-1629
Fax: (603) 225-1580

Providence Area Office
Federal Office Building
380 Westminster Mall, Room 543
Providence, Rhode Island 02903
(401) 528-4669
Fax: (401) 528-4663

◆**Region 2**

Regional Office
201 Varick Street, Room 670
New York, New York 10014
(212) 337-2378
(212) 337-2371 FAX

Area Offices
New Jersey | New York | Puerto Rico| Virgin Islands

Avenel Area Office
1030 St. Georges Avenue
Plaza 35, Suite 205
Avenel, New Jersey 07001
(732) 750-3270
(732) 750-4737 FAX

Hasbrouck Heights Area Office
500 Route 17 South
2nd Floor
Hasbrouck Heights, New Jersey 07604
(201) 288-1700
(201) 288-7315 FAX

Marlton Area Office
Marlton Executive Park, Building 2
701 Route 73 South, Suite 120
Marlton, New Jersey 08053
(856) 396-2594
(856) 396-2593 FAX

Parsippany Area Office
299 Cherry Hill Road, Suite 103
Parsippany, New Jersey 07054
(973) 263-1003
(973) 299-7161 FAX

Albany Area Office
401 New Karner Road, Suite 300
Albany, New York 12205-3809
(518) 464-4338
(518) 464-4337 FAX

Queens District Office of the Manhattan Area Office
45-17 Marathon Parkway
Little Neck, NY 11362
(718) 279-9060
(718) 279-9057 FAX

Buffalo Area Office
U. S. Dept. of Labor/OSHA
130 S. Elmwood Avenue, Suite 500
Buffalo, NY 14202-2465
(716) 551-3053
(716) 551-3126 FAX

Long Island Area Office
1400 Old Country Road
Suite 208
Westbury, New York 11590
(516) 334-3344
(516) 334-3326 FAX

Manhattan Area Office
201 Varick Street RM. 908
New York, NY 10014
(212) 620-3200
(212) 620-4121 (FAX)

Syracuse Area Office
3300 Vickery Road
North Syracuse, New York 13212
(315) 451-0808
(315) 451-1351 FAX

Tarrytown Area Office
660 White Plains Road, 4th Floor
Tarrytown, New York 10591-5107
(914) 524-7510
(914) 524-7515 FAX

Puerto Rico Area Office
Triple S Building
1510 FD Roosevelt Avenue, Suite 5B
Guaynabo, Puerto Rico 00968
(787) 277-1560
(787) 277-1567 FAX

◆**Region 3**

Regional Office
U.S. Department of Labor/OSHA
The Curtis Center-Suite 740 West
170 S. Independence Mall West
Philadelphia, PA 19106-3309
TELE: (215) 861-4900
FAX: (215) 861-4904

Area Offices
District of Columbia | Delaware | Maryland | Pennsylvania | Virginia |
West Virginia

Baltimore/Washington D.C. Area Office
OSHA Area Office
U.S. Department of Labor-OSHA
1099 Winterson Road, Suite 140
Linthicum, Maryland 21090
Phone: (410) 865-2055/2056
(410) 865-2068 FAX

Wilmington Area Office
Mellon Bank Building, Suite 900
919 Market Street
Wilmington, Delaware 19801-3319
(302) 573-6518
(302) 573-6532 FAX

Baltimore/Washington D.C. Area Office
OSHA Area Office
U.S. Department of Labor-OSHA
1099 Winterson Road, Suite 140
Linthicum, Maryland 21090
Phone: (410) 865-2055/2056
Fax: (410) 865-2068

Allentown Area Office
850 North 5th Street
Allentown, Pennsylvania 18102
(610) 776-0592
(610) 776-1913 FAX

Erie Area Office
1128 State Street, Suite 200
Erie, Pennsylvania 16501
(814) 461-1492
(814) 461-1498 FAX

Harrisburg Area Office
Progress Plaza
49 North Progress Avenue
Harrisburg, Pennsylvania 17109-3596
(717) 782-3902
(717) 782-3746 FAX

Philadelphia Area Office
US Custom House, Room 242
Second & Chestnut Street
Philadelphia, Pennsylvania 19106-2902
(215) 597-4955
(215) 597-1956 FAX

Pittsburgh Area Office
U.S. Department of Labor-OSHA
William Moorhead Federal Building, Room 905
1000 Liberty Avenue
Pittsburgh, PA 15222
(412) 395-4903
(412) 395-6380 FAX

Wilkes-Barre Area Office
The Stegmaier Building, Suite 410
7 North Wilkes-Barre Boulevard
Wilkes-Barre, PA 18702-5241
(570) 826-6538
(570) 821-4170 FAX

Norfolk Area Office
Federal Office Building, Room 614
200 Granby Street
Norfolk, Virginia 23510-1811
(757) 441-3820
(No direct lines to staff)
(757) 441-3594 FAX

Charleston Area Office
405 Capitol Street, Suite 407
Charleston, West Virginia 25301-1727
(304) 347-5937
(No direct lines to staff)
(304) 347-5275 FAX

◆ **Region 4**

Regional Office
61 Forsyth Street, SW
Room 6T50
Atlanta, Georgia 30303
(404) 562-2300
(404) 562-2295 FAX

Area Offices
Alabama | Florida | Georgia | Kentucky | Mississippi | North Carolina |
South Carolina | Tennessee

Birmingham Area Office
Medical Forum Building
950 22nd Street North, Room 1500
Birmingham, AL 35203
(205) 731-1534
(205) 731-0504 FAX

Mobile Area Office
1141 Montlimar Drive, Suite 1006
Mobile Alabama 36609
(251) 441-6131
(251) 441-6396 FAX

Fort Lauderdale Area Office
8040 Peters Road, Building H-100
Fort Lauderdale, Florida 33324
(954) 424-0242
(954) 424-3073 FAX

Jacksonville Area Office
Ribault Building, Suite 227
1851 Executive Center Drive
Jacksonville, Florida 32207
(904) 232-2895
(904) 232-1294 FAX

Tampa Area Office
5807 Breckenridge Parkway, Suite A
Tampa, Florida 33610-4249
(813) 626-1177
(813) 626-7015 FAX

Atlanta East Area Office
LaVista Perimeter Office Park
2183 N. Lake Parkway, Building 7
Suite 110
Tucker, Georgia 30084-4154
(770) 493-6644
(770) 493-7725 FAX

Atlanta West Area Office
2400 Herodian Way, Suite 250
Smyrna, Georgia 30080-2968
(770) 984-8700
(770) 984-8855 FAX

Savannah Area Office
450 Mall Boulevard, Suite J
Savannah, Georgia 31406
(912) 652-4393
(912) 652-4329 FAX

Frankfort Area Office
John C. Watts Federal Office Building
330 West Broadway, Room 108
Frankfort, Kentucky 40601-1922
(502) 227-7024
(502) 227-2348 FAX

Jackson Area Office
3780 I-55 North, Suite 210
Jackson, Mississippi 39211-6323
(601) 965-4606
(601) 965-4610 FAX

Raleigh Area Office
4407 Bland Road
Somerset Park Suite 210
Raleigh, North Carolina 27609
(919) 790-8096
(919) 790-8224 FAX

Columbia Area Office
Strom Thurmond Federal Building
1835 Assembly Street, Room 1472
Columbia, South Carolina 29201-2453
(803) 765-5904
(803) 765-5591 FAX

Nashville Area Office
51 Century Boulevard Suite 340,
Nashville, TN 37214
(615) 232-3803
(615) 232-3827 FAX

◆ Region 5

Regional Office
230 South Dearborn Street, Room 3244
Chicago, Illinois 60604
(312) 353-2220
(312) 353-7774 FAX

Area Offices
Illinois | Indiana | Michigan | Minnesota | Ohio | Wisconsin
Calumet City Area Office

1600 167th Street, Suite 9
Calumet City, Illinois 60409
(708) 891-3800
(708) 862-9659 FAX

Chicago North Area Office
701 Lee Street - Suite 950
Des Plaines, Illinois 60016
(847) 803-4800
(847) 390-8220 FAX

Fairview Heights District Office
11 Executive Drive, Suite 11
Fairview Heights, Illinois 62208
(618) 632-8612
(618) 632-5712 FAX

North Aurora Area Office
365 Smoke Tree Plaza
North Aurora, IL 60542
(630) 896-8700
(630) 892-2160 FAX

Peoria Area Office
2918 W. Willows Knolls Road
Peoria, Illinois 61614
(309) 589-7033
(309) 589-7326 FAX

Indianapolis Area Office
46 East Ohio Street, Room 453
Indianapolis, Indiana 46204
(317) 226-7290
(317) 226-7292 FAX

Lansing Area Office
U.S. Department of Labor
Occupational Safety and Health Administration
315 West Allegan Street, Suite 207
Lansing, Michigan 48933
(517) 487-4996
(517) 487-4997 FAX

Eau Claire Area Office
1310 W. Clairemont Avenue
Eau Claire, Wisconsin 54701
(715) 832-9019
(715) 832-1147 FAX

Cincinnati Area Office
36 Triangle Park Drive
Cincinnati, Ohio 45246
(513) 841-4132
(513) 841-4114 FAX

Cleveland Area Office
1240 East 9th Street, Room 899
Cleveland, Ohio 44199
(216) 615-4266
(216) 615-4234 FAX

Columbus Area Office
200 North High Street, Room 620
Columbus, Ohio 43215
(614) 469-5582
(614) 469-6791 FAX

Toledo Area Office
420 Madison Avenue, Suite 600
Toledo, Ohio 43604
(419) 259-7542
(419) 259-6355 FAX

Appleton Area Office
1648 Tri Park Way
Appleton, Wisconsin 54914
(920) 734-4521
(920) 734-2661 FAX

Madison Area Office
4802 E. Broadway
Madison, Wisconsin 53716
(608) 441-5388
(608) 441-5400 FAX

Milwaukee Area Office
310 West Wisconsin Avenue, Room 1180
Milwaukee, Wisconsin 53203
(414) 297-3315
(414) 297-4299 FAX

◆**Region 6**

Regional Office
525 Griffin Street, Suite 602
Dallas, Texas 75202
(972) 850-4145
(972) 850-4149 FAX
(972) 850-4150 FSO FAX

Area Offices
Arkansas | Louisiana | New Mexico | Oklahoma | Texas
Little Rock Area Office
10810 Executive Center Dr
Danville Bldg #2; Ste 206
Little Rock, AR 72211
Phone 501-224-1841
Fax 501-224-4431

Baton Rouge Area Office
9100 Bluebonnet Centre Blvd, Suite 201
Baton Rouge, Louisiana 70809
(225) 298-5458
(225) 298-5457 FAX

Lubbock Area Office
1205 Texas Avenue, Room 806
Lubbock, Texas 79401
(806) 472-7681
(806) 472-7686 FAX

Oklahoma City Area Office
55 North Robinson - Suite 315
Oklahoma City, Oklahoma 73102-9237
(405) 278-9560
(405) 278-9572 FAX

Austin Area Office
La Costa Green Bldg.,
1033 La Posada Dr. Suite 375
Austin, Texas 78752-3832
(512) 374-0271
(512) 374-0086 FAX

Corpus Christi Area Office
Wilson Plaza
606 N Carancahua, Ste. 700
Corpus Christi, Texas 78476
(361) 888-3420
(361) 888-3424 FAX

Dallas Area Office
8344 East RL Thornton Freeway
Suite 420
Dallas, Texas 75228
(214) 320-2400
(214) 320–2598 FAX

El Paso District Office
U.S. Dept. of Labor - OSHA
4849 N. Mesa, Suite 200
El Paso, TX 79912-5936
(915) 534-6251
(915) 534-6259 FAX

Fort Worth Area Office
North Starr II, Suite 302
8713 Airport Freeway
Fort Worth, Texas 76180-7610
(817) 428-2470
(817) 581-7723 FAX

Houston North Area Office
507 North Sam Houston Parkway East
Suite 400
Houston, Texas 77060
(281) 591-2438
(281) 999-7457 FAX

Houston South Area Office
17625 El Camino Real, Suite 400
Houston, Texas 77058
(281) 286-0583
(281) 286-6352 FAX
Toll Free: (800) 692-4202

Lubbock Area Office
1205 Texas Avenue, Room 806
Lubbock, Texas 79401
(806) 472-7681 (7685)
(806) 472-7686 FAX

San Antonio District Office
Washington Square Blvd, Suite 203
800 Dolorosa Street
San Antonio, TX 78207-4559
(210) 472-5040
(210) 472-5045 FAX

◆ **Region 7**

Regional Office
Two Pershing Square Building
2300 Main Street, Suite 1010
Kansas City, Missouri 64108-2416
Phone: (816) 283-8745
Voice: (816) 283-0545
FAX: (816) 283-0547

Area Offices
Iowa | Kansas | Missouri | Nebraska

U.S. Department of Labor
Occupational Safety and Health Administration
210 Walnut ST RM 815
Des Moines IA 50309-2015
(515) 284-4794
(515) 284-4058 FAX

Wichita Area Office
271 W. 3rd Street North, Room 400
Wichita, KS 67202
(316) 269-6644
(316) 269-6646 Voice Mail
(316) 269-6185 FAX
Toll Free (Kansas Residents Only): 1-800-362-2896

Kansas City Area Office
2300 Main Street, Suite 168
Kansas City, Missouri 64108
(816) 483-9531
(816) 483-9724 Fax
Toll Free (Missouri Residents Only): 1-800-892-2674

St. Louis Area Office
1222 Spruce Street, Room 9.104
St. Louis, Missouri 63103
(314) 425-4249
(314) 425-4255 Voice Mail
(314) 425-4289 Fax
Toll Free (Missouri Residents Only): 1-800-392-7743

Omaha Area Office
Overland-Wolf Building
6910 Pacific Street, Room 100
Omaha, Nebraska 68106
(402) 553-0171
(402) 551-1288 FAX
Toll Free (Nebraska Residents Only): 1-800-642-8963

◆Region 8

Regional Office
1999 Broadway, Suite 1690
Denver, Colorado 80202
720-264-6550
720-264-6585 FAX

Area Offices
Colorado | Montana | North Dakota | South Dakota

Denver Area Office
1391 Speer Boulevard, Suite 210
Denver, Colorado 80204-2552
(303) 844-5285
(303) 844-6676 FAX

The Denver Area Office also oversees the federal program for Utah. Contact: Herb Gibson, Area Director, Denver Area Office, (303) 844-5285, Ext. 106.

Englewood Area Office
7935 East Prentice Avenue, Suite 209
Englewood, Colorado 80111-2714
(303) 843-4500
(303) 843-4515 FAX

Billings Area Office
2900 4th Avenue North, Suite 303
Billings, Montana 59101
(406) 247-7494
(406) 247-7499 FAX

Bismarck Area Office
Federal Office Building
1640 East Capitol Avenue
Bismarck, North Dakota 58501
(701) 250-4521
(701) 250-4520 FAX

Bruce Beelman, Area Director
U.S. Department of Labor
Occupational Safety and Health Administration
Bismarck Area Office
1640 East Capitol Avenue
Bismarck, ND 58501
(701) 250-4521

◆Region 9

Region IX Federal Contact Numbers
90 7th Street, Suite 18100
San Francisco, California 94103
(415) 625-2547
For Arizona, California, Guam, Hawaii, and Nevada

◆Region 10

Regional Office
1111 Third Avenue, Suite 715
Seattle, Washington 98101-3212
(206) 553-5930
(206) 553-6499 FAX

Area Offices
Alaska | Idaho | Oregon | Washington

Anchorage Area Office
Scott Ketcham, Area Director
U.S. Department of Labor - OSHA
222 W. 7th Avenue, Box 22
Anchorage, AK 99513
Comm. Phone: (907) 271-5152
Facsimile Number: (907) 271-4238

Boise Area Office
1150 North Curtis Road, Suite 201
Boise, Idaho 83706
(208) 321-2960
(208) 321-2966 Fax

Portland Area Office
Federal Office Building
1220 Southwest 3rd Avenue, Room 640
Portland, Oregon 97204
(503) 326-2251
(503) 326-3574 FAX

Bellevue Area Office
505 106th Avenue NE, Suite 302
Bellevue, Washington 98004
Comm. Phone: (425) 450-5480
Facsimile Number: (425) 450-5483

NFPA 70E FREQUENTLY ASKED QUESTIONS

Q. *How do I determine what level of protection I need for my job task?*

A. First, reference Table 130.7(C)(9)(a) of the NFPA 70E 2009 edition. This will determine the hazard category of your job task (0-4). Second, consult Reference Table 130.7(C)(10) of the standard to determine what clothing and equipment is required based on the hazard/risk category that was determined. Third, Reference Table 130.7(C)(11) will determine what ATPV rating is necessary. Once you have determined the ATPV rating, simply find the ATPV rating on the garment (required on tag) that meets or exceeds your requirement.

Q. *What if my job task is not listed in Table 130.7(C)(9)(a) of NFPA 70E Standard?*

A. A flash hazard analysis must be done. The Duke Power Flux Calculator meets this requirement.

Q. *Is Compliance with NFPA 70E mandatory?*

A. No, NFPA 70E is a national consensus safety standard published by NFPA primarily to assist OSHA in preparing electrical safety standards. Federal OSHA has not incorporated it into the Code of Federal Regulations.

Q. *Can I be cited for not complying with NFPA 70E?*

A. Yes, the employer must assess the workplace for electrical hazards and the need for PPE under 29CFR 1910.335(a)(1)(i). Details on how to comply with this standard is up to the employer. The employer is expected to use the best means available to comply with this requirement, and that is done through consensus standard NFPA 70E. Compliance with 70E will assure compliance with this OSHA requirement. In the event of an injury or death due to an electrical accident, if OSHA determines that compliance with 70E would have prevented or lessened the injury, OSHA may cite the employer under the general duty clause. In 2003 "Standards Interpretation" letter OSHA stated 70E can be used as evidence of whether the employer acted reasonably.

TABLE 130.7 (C)(11) Protective Clothing Characteristics

Hazard/Risk Category	Clothing Description	APTV Rating Cal/cm2
0	Untreated Cotton, Wool, Rayon, Silk, or Blend. Fabric weight >4.5oz/Yd2 (1 layer)	N/A
1	FR Shirt and FR Pants or FR Coverall (1 layer)	4
2	Cotton underwear plus FR shirt and FR pants (1 or 2 layers)	8
3	Cotton underwear plus FR shirt and FR pants plus FR coverall, cotton underwear plus two FR Coveralls (2 or 3 layers)	25
4	Cotton underwear plus FR shirt and FR pants plus multi-layer flash suit (3 or more layers)	40

<u>PPE TABLE</u>

Hazard/Risk Category Classification (within flash protection boundary)

Low-voltage tasks (600 volts and below), chart applies when there is an available short-circuit capacity of 25 kA or less, and when the fault clearing time is 0.03 seconds (2 cycles) or less.
For 600-volt-class motor control centers, a short-circuit current capacity of 65 kA or less and fault-clearing time of 0.33 seconds (20 cycles) is permitted.
For 600-volt-class switchgear, a short-circuit current capacity of 65 kA or less and fault-clearing time of 1 seconds (60 cycles) is used.

TASK:	PPE Category	V-R Gloves	V-R Tools
Opening Doors and Covers			
Open hinged covers (to expose bare, energized parts)			
240 volts or less	0	N	N
600-volt-class motor control centers	1	N	N
600-volt-class lighting or small power transformers	1	N	N
600-volt-class switchgear (with power circuit breakers or fused switches)	2	N	N
NEMA E2 (fused contactor) motor starters, 2.3 kV through 7.2 kV	3	N	N
1 kV and over (metal clad switchgear)	3	N	N
1 kV and higher, (metal clad load interrupter switches, fused or unfused)	3	N	N
Remove bolted covers (expose bare, energized parts)			
240 volts or less	1	N	N
600-volt-class motor control centers or transformers	2*	N	N
600-volt-class lighting or small power transformers	2*	N	N
600-volt-class switchgear (with power circuit breakers or fused switches)	3	N	N
NEMA E2 (fused contactor) motor starters, 2.3 kV through 7.2 kV	4	N	N
1 kV and higher (metal clad switchgear)	4	N	N
1 kV and higher, (metal clad load interrupter switches, fused or unfused)	4	N	N
Open transformer compartments (metal clad switchgear 1 kV and higher)	4	N	N

Installing, Removing, Operating: Circuit Breakers (CBs), Fused Switches, Motors Starters or Fused Contactors			
Installing or removing circuit breakers or fused switches, 240 volts or less	**1**	Y	Y
Insert or remove (rack) CBs from cubicles, doors closed			
600-volt switchgear (with power circuit breakers or fused switches)	**2**	N	N
NEMA E2 (fused contactor) motor starters, 2.3 kV through 7.2 kV	**2**	N	N
1 kV and higher (metal clad switchgear)	**2**	N	N
Insert or remove (rack) CBs or starters from cubicles, doors open			
600-volt-class switchgear (with power circuit breakers or fused switches)	**3**	N	N
NEMA E2 (fused contactor) Motor Starters, 2.3 kV through 7.2 kV	**3**	N	N
1 kV and higher (metal clad switchgear)	**4**	N	N
Operate circuit breaker (CB), fused switch, motor starter or fused contactor- covers on, doors closed			
240 volts or less	**0**	N	N
Over 240 but less than 600 volts panelboards	**0**	N	N
600 volts class motor control centers	**0**	N	N
600 volts class switchgear (with power circuit breakers or fused switches)	**0**	N	N
NEMA E2 (fused contactor) motor starters, 2.3 kV through 7.2 kV	**0**	N	N
1 kV and higher (metal clad switchgear)	**2**	N	N
1 kV and higher (metal clad load interrupter switches, fused or unfused)	**2**	N	N
Operate circuit breaker (CB), fused switch, motor starter or fused contactor-covers off, doors open			
240 volts or less	**0**	N	N
Over 240 but less than 600 volts panelboards	**1**	N	N
600 volts class motor control centers	**1**	N	N
600 volts class switchgear (with power circuit breakers or fused switches)	**1**	N	N
NEMA E2 (fused contactor) motor starters, 2.3 kV through 7.2 kV	**2***	N	N
1 kV and higher (metal clad switchgear)	**4**	N	N
2* = A double-layer switching hood and hearing protection are required, in addition to the other hazard/risk category 2 requirements of table 3-3.9.2 of Part II of NFPA 70E.			

TASK:	PPE Category	V-R Gloves	V-R Tools
Work on Energized Parts			
Work on energized parts, voltage testing, applying safety grounds			
240 volts or less	1	Y	Y
Over 240 but less than 600 volts panelboards	2*	Y	Y
600-volt-class motor control centers	2*	Y	Y
600-volt-class switchgear (with power circuit breakers or fused switches)	2*	Y	Y
600-volt-class lighting or small power transformers	2*	Y	Y
600-volt-class revenue meters	2*	Y	Y
NEMA E2 (fused contactor) motor starters, 2.3 kV through 7.2 kV	3	Y	Y
1 kV and higher (metal clad switchgear)	4	Y	Y
1 kV and higher metal clad load interrupter switches, fused or unfused	4	Y	Y
Work on control circuits with exposed energized parts, 120 volts or below			
600-volt-class motor control centers	0	Y	Y
600-volt-class switchgear (with power circuit breakers or fused switches)	0	Y	Y
NEMA E2 (fused contactor) motor starters, 2.3 kV through 7.2 kV	0	Y	Y
1 kV and higher (metal clad switchgear)	2	Y	Y
Work on control circuits with exposed energized parts, over 120 volts			
600-volt-class motor control centers	2*	Y	Y
600-volt-class switchgear (with power circuit breakers or fused switches)	2*	Y	Y
NEMA E2 (fused contactor) motor starters, 2.3 kV through 7.2 kV	3	Y	Y
1 kV and higher (metal clad switchgear)	4	Y	Y

2* = A double-layer switching hood and hearing protection are required, in addition to the other hazard/risk category 2 requirements of table 3-3.9.2 of Part II of NFPA 70E.

Applying safety grounds after voltage testing does not require voltage-rated tools. Voltage-rated gloves or tools are rated and tested for the maximum line-to-line voltage on which work will be done. The hazard/risk category may be reduced by one number for low-voltage equipment listed here where the short-circuit current available is less than 15 kA (less than 25 kA for 600-volt-class switchgear).

PPE CLOTHES SELECTION CHART

WORK/TASK	CLOTHING TO WEAR
All hazard/risk category 1 and 2 tasks Systems operating at less than 1000 volts, these tasks include work on all equipment *except* • Insertion/removal of low-voltage motor starter "buckets" • Insertion/removal of power circuit breakers with the switchgear doors open • Removal of bolted covers from switchgear. On systems operating at 1000 volts or more, tasks also include the operation, insertion, or removal of switching devices *with equipment enclosure doors closed.*	**Everyday work clothing** Flame-resistant long-sleeve shirt (minimum ATPV of 5) <u>worn over</u> an untreated cotton T-shirt with <u>FR pants</u> (minimum ATPV of 8) *Or* FR coveralls (minimum ATPV of 5) <u>worn over</u> an untreated cotton T-shirt (or an untreated natural-fiber long-sleeve shirt) with untreated natural-fiber pants.
All hazard/risk category 3 and 4 tasks listed in table 2 On systems operating at 1000 volts or more, these tasks include work on energized parts of all equipment. On systems of less than 1000 volts, tasks include insertion or removal of low-voltage motor-start motor control center "buckets," insertion or removal of power circuit breakers with the switchgear enclosure doors open, and removal of bolted covers from switchgear.	**Electric "switching" clothing** Double-layer FR flash jacket and FR bib overalls <u>worn over</u> either FR coveralls (minimum ATPV of 5) or FR long-sleeve shirt and FR pants (minimum ATPV of 5) <u>worn over</u> untreated natural-fiber long-sleeve shirt and pants <u>worn over</u> an untreated cotton T-shirt *Or* Insulated FR coveralls (minimum ATPV of 25, independent of other layers) <u>worn over</u> untreated natural-fiber long-sleeve shirt with untreated cotton blue jeans ("regular weight," minimum 12 oz./sq. yd. fabric weight), <u>worn over</u> an untreated cotton T-shirt.

SAMPLE SIMPLE LOCKOUT/TAGOUT WORK PLAN

Job Name: _____   Start Date: _____   End Date: _____

Site Location: _____   Qualified Worker: _____

SCOPE OF WORK:

1. Description of circuit/equipment to be locked out: _____
_____

2. Description of work to be done: _____
_____

3. Lists types and voltage of energy source: _____
_____

De-energizing Equipment to Service

1) Method to dissipate or restrain stored energy: _____ (electrical/capacitors – grounding; springs/elevated machines-blocking; hydraulic/pneumatic – bleeding)

2) Notify all Affected Employees/Workers (persons in the area of the equipment and operators of equipment)

3) Apply your lock to the disconnecting device.

4) Verify equipment is disconnected by testing to ensure that the equipment will not operate. If controls are operated to check disconnection, return operating controls to neutral or off position. **NOTE:** Make sure no workers will be exposed during this step

Restoring Equipment to Service

1) Check area that tools & nonessential items removed

2) Check all guards and covers installed properly

3) Check that all controls are in neutral position

4) Check that all personnel are safely positioned

5) Remove lockout devices and notify Affected Employees/Workers that work is complete and equipment is ready for use.

JOB SAFETY ANALYSIS FORM

JOB SAFETY ANALYSIS		Date:

Prepared by:	Project Address:	Emergency Contact Person:
		Emergency Phone Numbers:
Specific Work Location(s):		Prejob Walkthrough Conducted: ☐ Yes ☐ No

Work Scope/Description:

KNOWN OR POTENTIAL HAZARDS

		Yes	No	Reference			Yes	No	Reference
1. Lock and Tag	☒ ⊕ ☑	☐	☐	29 CFR 1910.147	8. Electrical Hazards ☒ ⊕ ☑		☐	☐	29CFR1926 Subpart K NFPA 70E
2. Hot Work	☒ ⊕ ☑	☐	☐	29CFR1926 Subpart F & J	9. Hazardous Materials ☒		☐	☐	29CFR1926.59
Qualified Person:									
3. Fall Hazards (>6 ft)	☒ ☑	☐	☐	29CFR1926 Subpart M	☒ = Requires formal/special training				
4. Scaffolding	☒ ☑	☐	☐	29CFR1926 Subpart L	⊕ = Requires a permit/form/report				
5. Aerial Lifts	☒ ☑	☐	☐	29CFR1926 Subpart J	☑ = Requires certification or competent/qualified person designation				
6. Excavation/Trenching	⊕ ☑	☐	☐	29CFR1926 Subpart P	**10. MINIMUM DRESS/PPE REQUIREMENTS:** Substantial Footwear, Long Pants, Shirt with Sleeves, Hart Hat, Eye Protection				
7. Confined Space	☒ ⊕ ☑	☐	☐	29CFR1910 Subpart J	**ADDITIONAL PPE:**				

SPECIFIC HAZARD ANALYSIS AND SAFE WORK REQUIREMENTS

A detailed discussion of hazards specific to the work activity/location, including those noted above, has taken place. All workers are trained to perform the duties involved and safety controls have been identified.

ADDITIONAL TRAINING:

ACTIVITY AND SPECIFIC HAZARD	SAFE WORK REQUIREMENT/CONTROL

Index

Note: Page numbers followed by '*f*' indicate figures, '*b*' indicate boxes.

377

current-carrying conductors, 190, 193*f*
NEC 310.5, 190, 191*f*
requirements, 193–194
feeder and service loads
ampacity, 212
vs. branch-circuit loads, 209–210
calculations, 211–212
electric clothes dryer loads, 211
heating/cooling package unit, 207–208
lighting loads, 204–206
office heater loads, 206, 206*f*
Ohms law diagram, 207, 207*f*
quick reference electric motor load chart, 207, 208*f*
service disconnection, 212–213
small appliance and laundry loads, 210–211
feeder sizing
conductor amperage, 200
general-use receptacle, 202–203
grounding conductors, 201
lighting load, 203–204
load calculations, 201
OCPD, 199–200
protection, 200
flammable conditions
airborne environmental conditions, 50
air mixtures, 50–51
Article 501, 52
Article 502, 52
Article 503, Class III locations, 53
Class II, Division 1 location, 52
Class II, Division 2 location, 52–53
combustible dust environments, 51–52
fire prevention, 53
locations classifications, 49–50
overcurrent protection
circuit ampacity, 215, 215*f*
circuit breakers/fuses, 213–214, 214*f*
fault current, 213
generators, 216–218
motor circuit, 215, 216*f*
standard circuit breaker sizes, 214, 215*f*
transformers, 218
voltage rating, 213–214
National Electrical Safety Code (NESC®), 9
communication lines, 176–177
electric supply installations
conductors, 174–175
current and voltage transformers, 173–174
surge arresters, 175–176, 176*f*
grounded bus bars, 172, 173*f*

overhead power lines
line workers, 182, 183, 183*f*
power line spans, 178–180, 181*f*
structural clearance support, 183–184
supply employee safety, 180–182
power line safety, electricians
distance, equipment, 184, 186*f*
electrocution, 184, 185
energized power lines, 184, 185*f*
facts, potential hazards, 187–188, 188*f*
fallen power lines, 185–186, 187*f*
fiber optic cables, 186–187
safe clearances, 184
National Fire Protection Association (NFPA)
Board of Directors, 8
fire hazards, 47
minimum standards and requirements, 7
professional standard, 8
regulations development, 7
representatives, 8

O

Occupational Safety and Health Association (OSHA), 10–11, 11*f*, 38–39
bloodborne pathogens, 14
common workplace hazards, 13
confined space regulations
entry permit, 239
manholes, 237, 237*f*
"permit-required confined space"/"permit space", 237
posters, alert workers, 237, 238*f*
contestation, citation
authorization, negotiation, 247
OSHA hearing, 247–248, 249*f*
violation, 246–247
ergonomic injuries, 12–13
eye protection, 229–230, 231*f*
footwear, 236–237
frequent violation categories, 225–226
guards, 13
hardhat classifications
damaged hardhats, 234, 235*f*
hardhat manufacture, 234, 235*f*
three industrial classes, 233–234
head protection, 231–232
inspections, 239–246, 290, 291*f*
employees complaints and reports, 239–240, 241
inspection planning, 241–242
job supervisor, representative, 242–243, 244*f*
nightmare, standard violation, 244–246
opening meeting, 240

Printed in the United States
By Bookmasters